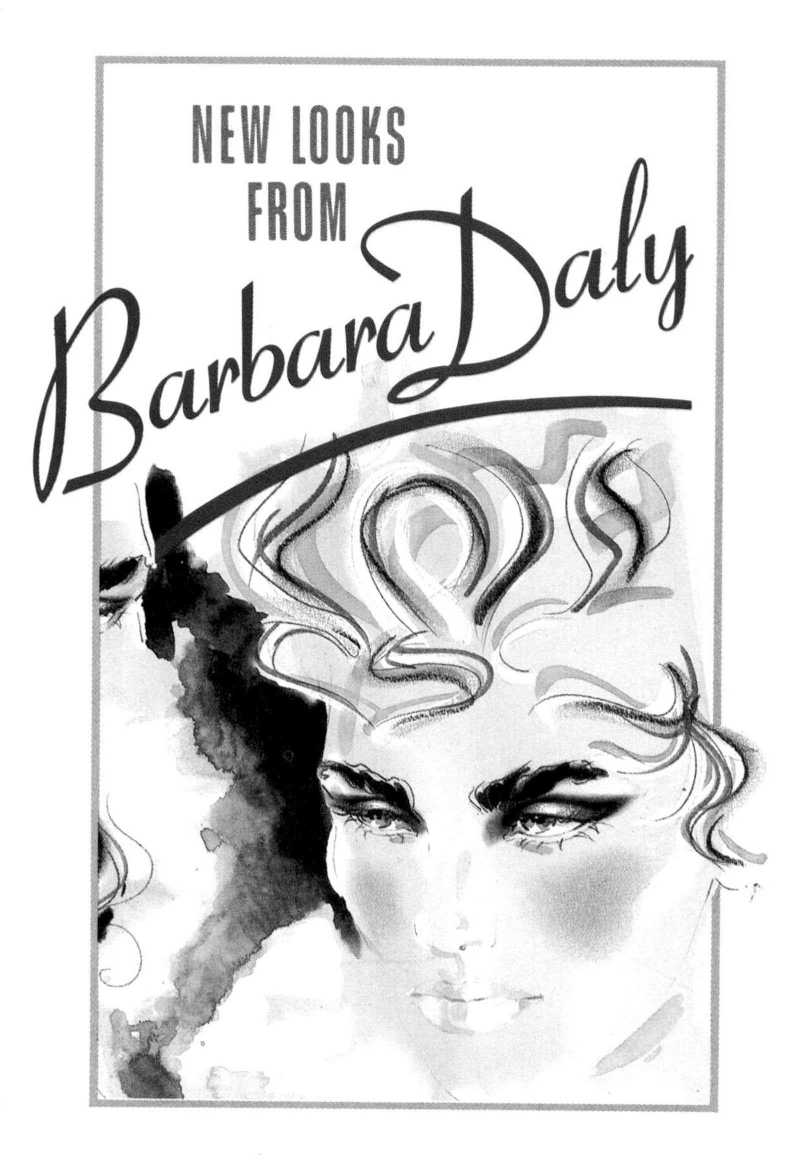
NEW LOOKS
FROM
Barbara Daly

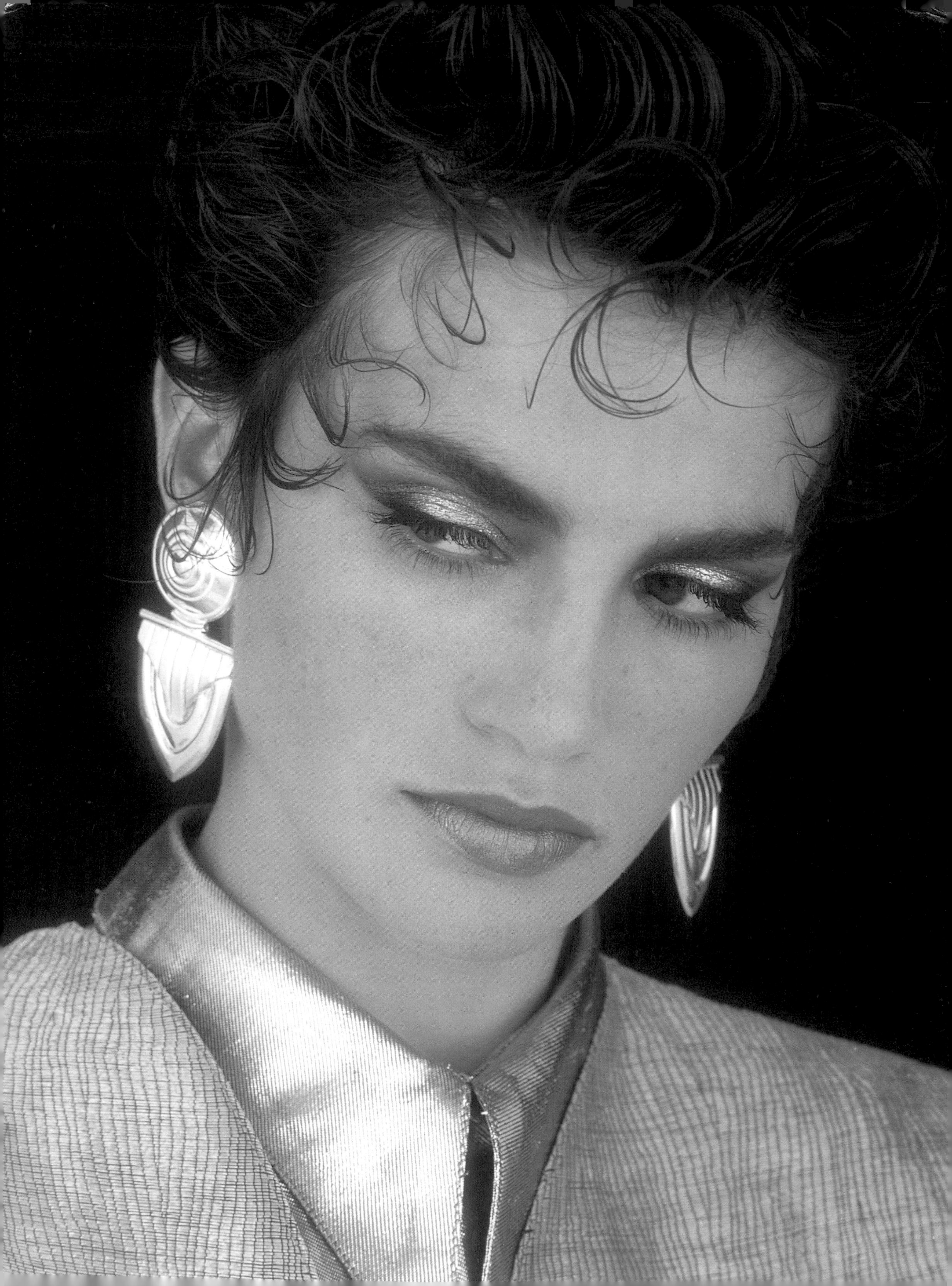

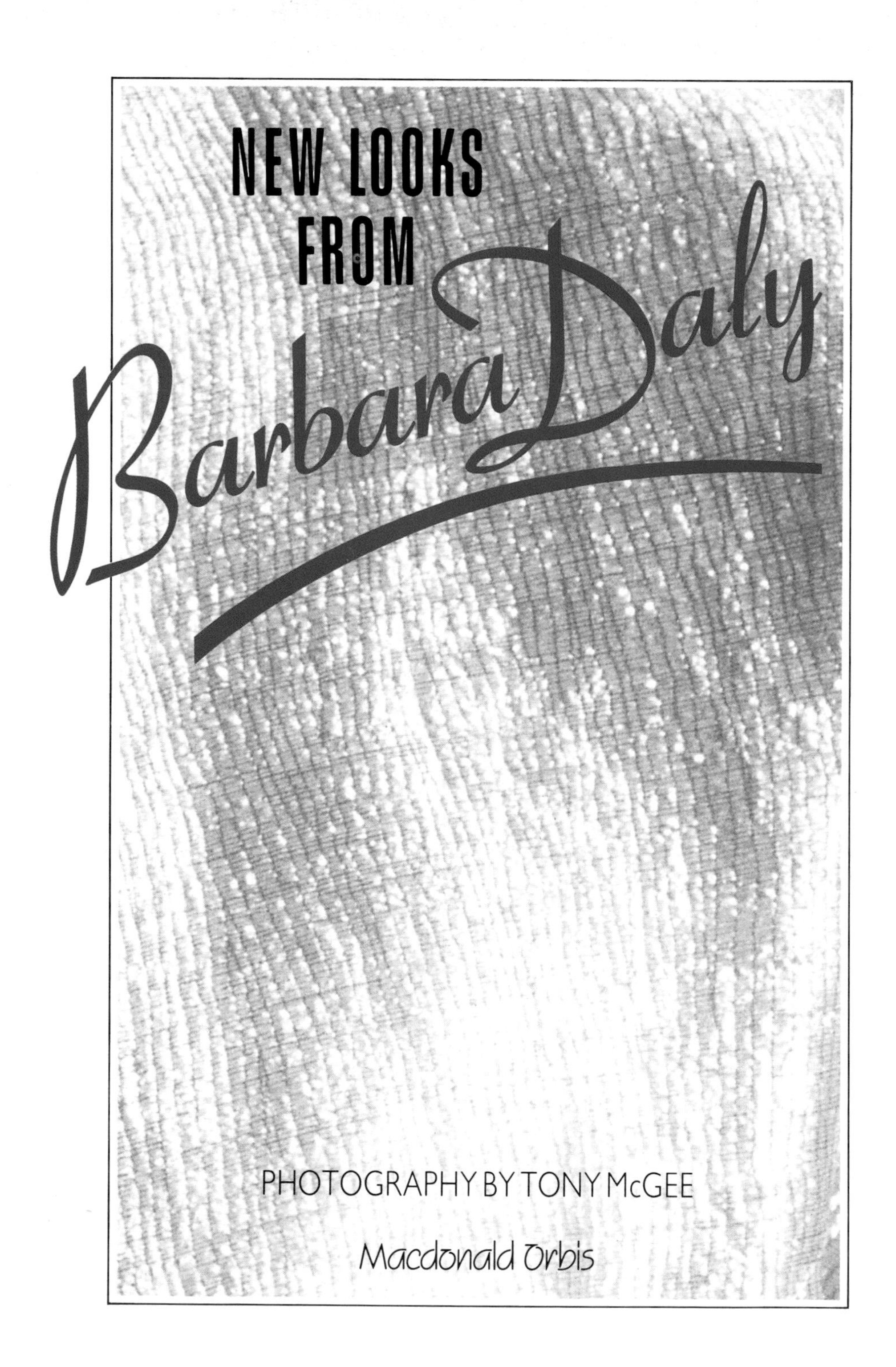

NEW LOOKS FROM Barbara Daly

PHOTOGRAPHY BY TONY McGEE

Macdonald Orbis

A Macdonald Orbis Book

For Laurence

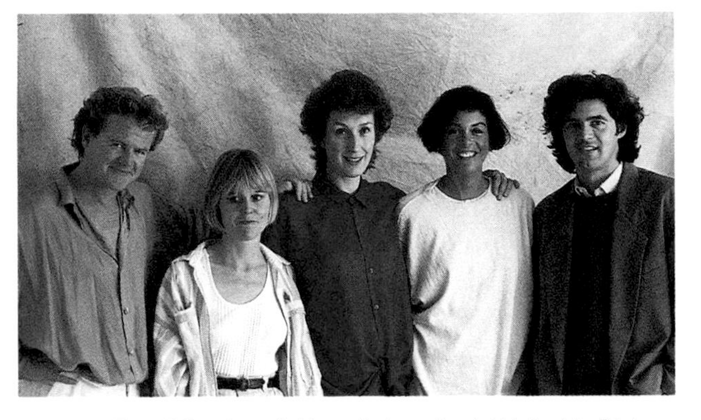

Left to right: Tony McGee · Lynne Robinson · Barbara · Annabel Hodin · John Frieda

Thank you
For special pictures to Tony McGee, to Lynne for wonderful drawings and to Paul Williams. To John Frieda and Nicky Clarke for contributing their immense talent and to 'mastermind' Annabel Hodin and Elspeth Norden for inspirational style. Thanks to Sarah, Mary, Suzy and Paul for their words, help and support, and last but not least, thank you to all the designers, without whose clothes, hats and jewellery the pages wouldn't have existed.

Love Barbara

Photography by Tony McGee

Styling by Annabel Hodin with Elspeth Norden

Hair by John Frieda and Nicky Clarke

Illustrations by Lynne Robinson

Still life photography by Paul Williams

First published in Great Britain in 1985 by Orbis Publishing Limited for Marks and Spencer plc.

This edition published in Great Britain in 1988 by Macdonald & Co (Publishers) Ltd.
London & Sydney

A Pergamon Press plc company

Colour separations by Imago Publishing
Printed by Novograph S.A., Spain

Notes on creating the hairstyles for *Colour Counsel* were written by John Frieda (J.F.)

Daly, Barbara
New looks from Barbara Daly.
1. Cosmetics 2. Face—Care and hygiene
I. Title
646.7'26'088042 RA778

ISBN 0-356-14410-0

Macdonald & Co (Publishers) Ltd
Greater London House
Hampstead Road
London NW1 7QX

CONTENTS

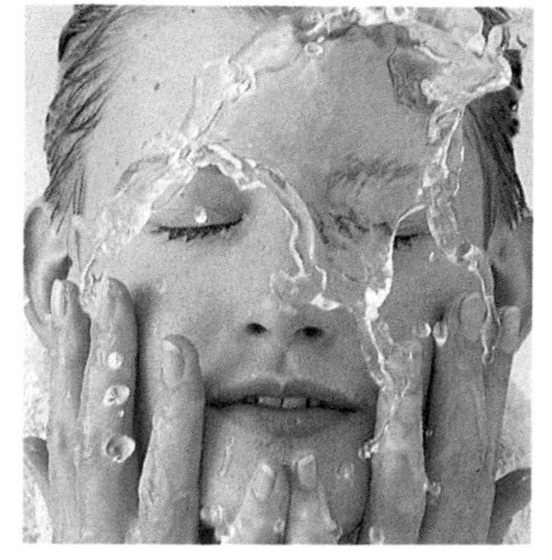

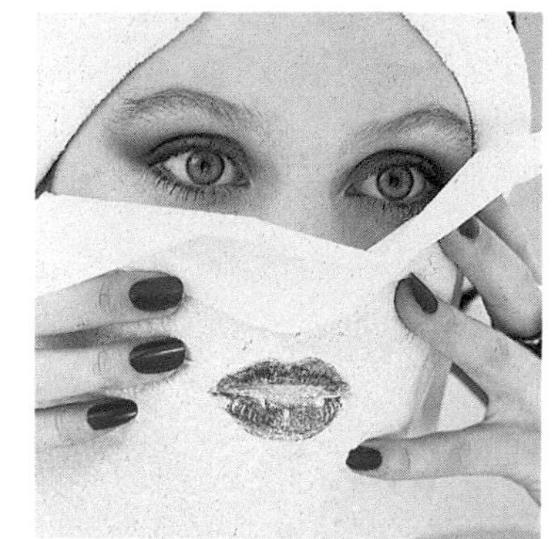

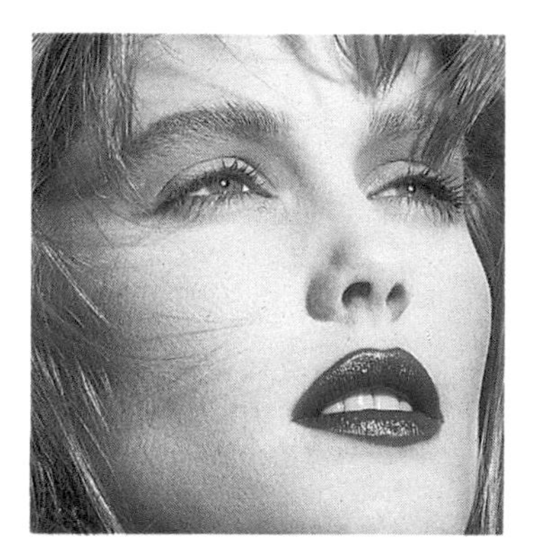

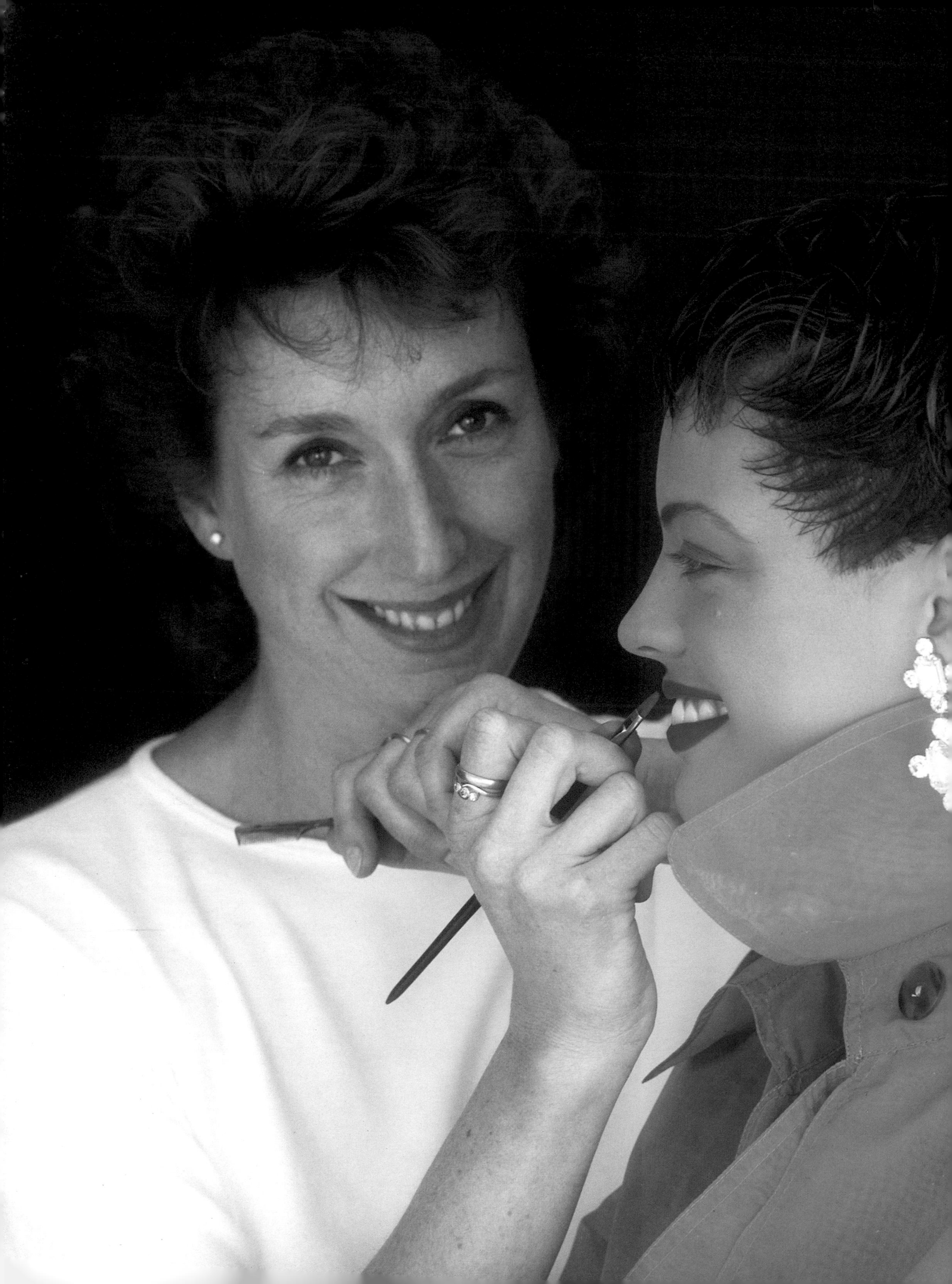

As a professional make-up artist, I am creating looks for today and for tomorrow. By presenting you with a whole book of new looks which break nearly every outdated colour rule, I hope to give you the enthusiasm to try something different for yourself.

Make-up is fashion. Even when you have found a look that is 'perfect' for you, it's a mistake never to change it, or it will soon start to date. I can often tell a woman's age quite precisely by the old-fashioned make-up she wears — a relic of her teenage years lovingly preserved. Sticking to the same tried-and-tested formula often degenerates into a quick five minutes in front of the mirror in a poor light because 'I could do it with my eyes closed'. The result does little for you; less than you deserve.

Make-up should involve experiment: spending time in front of the mirror trying out new colours and combinations. Keeping abreast of fashion doesn't mean going for an all-green face just because your favourite magazine says it's this month's look. It means not being afraid to try out new ideas and colours, and adapting them to your look, your personality, your clothes.

As well as new ideas, I am passing on to you the benefit of all my years of professional experience as a make-up artist. I tell you how to apply the make-up so that you have a superb, flawless finish, and I have included some of the secret tricks of my trade. Have fun!

Barbara Daly

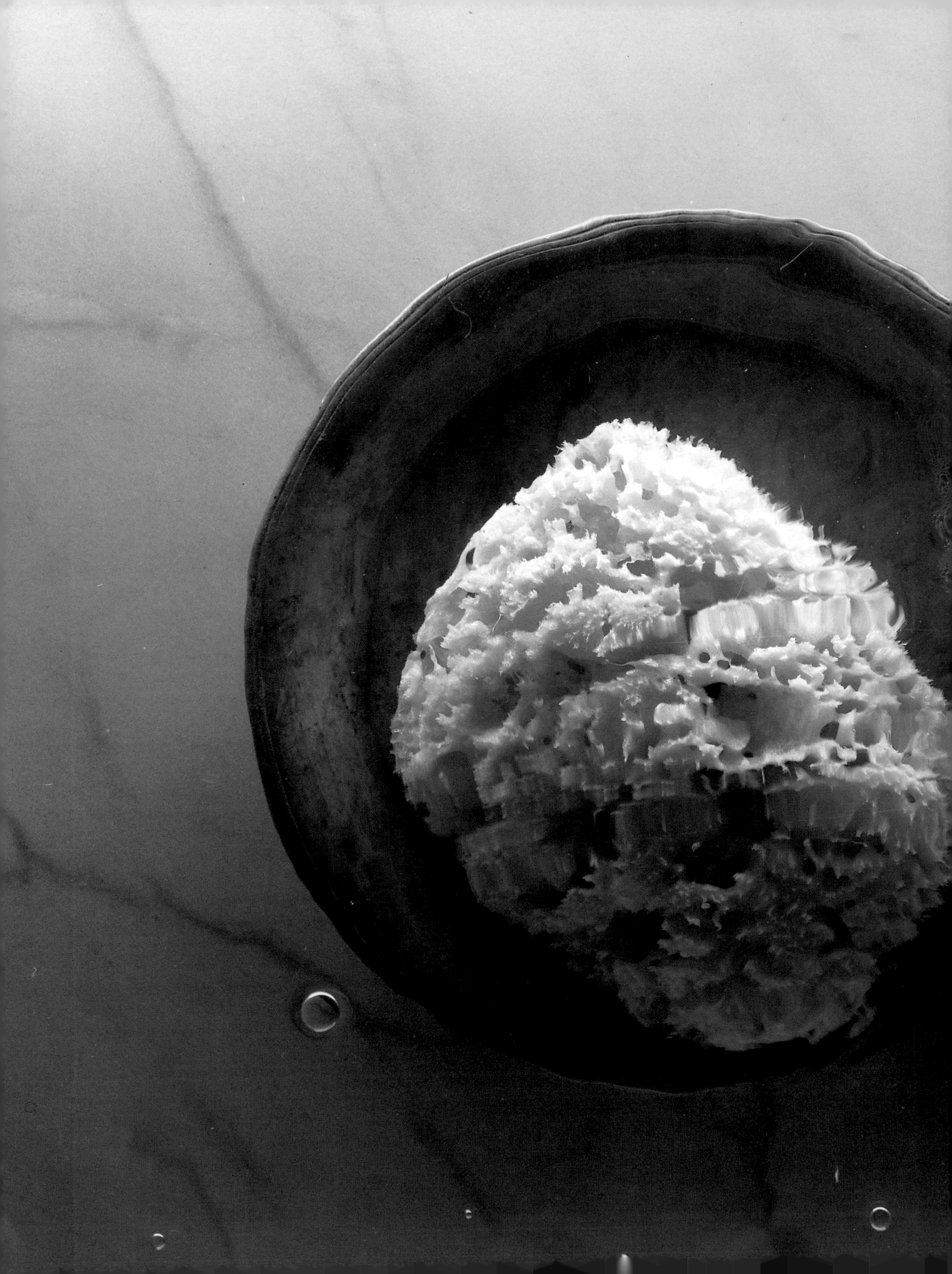

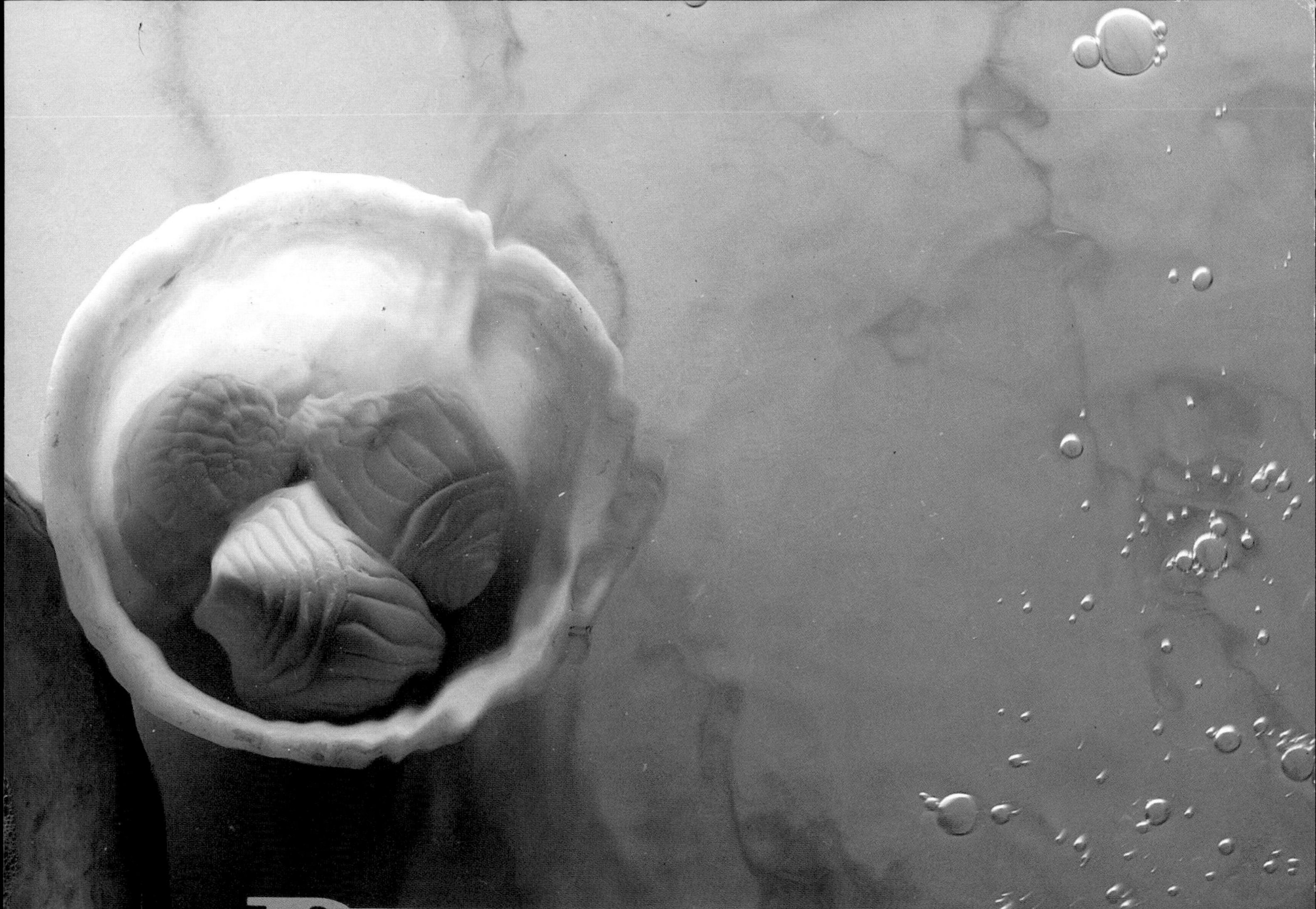

BEAUTY BASICS

Try as you may, beauty defies analysis: no particular feature, shape or colouring is a guarantee of it. But there is one thing that is recognized as a common attribute of beauty — lovely skin. A perfect skin is translucent, unblemished, with no dry or oily patches, silky-textured, and a smooth, even, all-over colour. Only the very few have perfect skin, and they were born with it. But good skin care can make up for much of what nature leaves out. There is no magic formula for perfect skin, but keeping to a simple daily routine and obeying just a few sensible rules enables you to make the very best of the skin you have — and is the only way to keep it youthful and glowing for the longest possible time.

Skin is quite tough by necessity. Just think of the job it has to do protecting your body! In return it deserves some loving care and attention. If you think that the very part you want to look the best – the skin on your face – is exposed all the time to the elements, it is understandable that even good skin can't be left to look after itself. Five minutes morning and night is all you need. Do so always and you'll keep a good skin good, and improve one that is less than perfect.

SKIN-CARE ROUTINE

There is no secret to looking after your skin, and no magic product that will instantly improve it. There are four basic steps to do every day: cleanse, moisturize, exfoliate and shield your skin from the sun.

CLEANSING

Skin must be cleansed twice a day, once in the morning and once at the end of the day before you go to bed, even if you don't wear make-up. Start at the collarbone and include your neck in your skin-care routine.

Choose a cream or milky cleanser recommended for your skin type, and use it to remove make-up and grime. Damp cotton wool is an efficient way to apply milky cleansers. Creamy cleansers, however, need to be massaged in gently with your fingertips before being wiped off with damp cotton wool. To remove the last traces of cleanser you can rinse with water, wash with a cleansing bar or mild soap, or use a toner. Toners can be too harsh for any but a very greasy or spotty skin. Remember, the less alcohol a toner contains the gentler it is. Deep cleansing, by steaming over a bowl of very hot water and using a cleansing face mask to draw out impurities, is good for all skins – once a month for greasy skins, every six to eight weeks for dry or sensitive skins.

MOISTURIZING

Skin needs moisturizer to stop water evaporating from the skin. Lack of moisture is one of the causes of wrinkles. You need to moisturize after cleansing morning and night, using the right product for your skin type.

EXFOLIATING

Exfoliation means using something mildly abrasive to clear the dead top layer of skin, make it look fresh and translucent and prepare it to absorb creams. On your face you can use exfoliating cream, washing grains, an abrasive puff, or natural ingredients such as oatmeal – as often as your skin needs it according to type.

PROTECTING FROM THE ELEMENTS

Moisturizer helps your skin in the battle against the drying effects of air-conditioning and heating, and the coarsening effect of wind, cold and rain. More care is needed to protect against the sun, which damages your skin permanently in the deepest layers where new skin is made, so that it ages more quickly. As the top layer of your skin renews itself completely every four weeks, even the best and deepest tan will fade within a month. You must decide if it is worth damaging your skin for ever for a few weeks of looking brown. If you do sunbathe then ration the time you spend in the sun and use a good sun cream, re-applied often. A high-factor sun blocking lotion will stop you burning, but it is still possible to tan slightly through it.

The products you choose to suit your skin vary according to your skin type, which I describe over the next four pages. Check which category your skin falls into. If it has elements of more than one, then you have combination skin, which is very common, and you should treat the dry and oily parts of your face separately with appropriate products.

Cleanliness is at the heart of every skin care routine. Even if you have very dry or sensitive skin you can allow yourself the refreshing sensation of water if you use a mild cleansing bar rather than soap and ensure that the water is only moderately lukewarm.

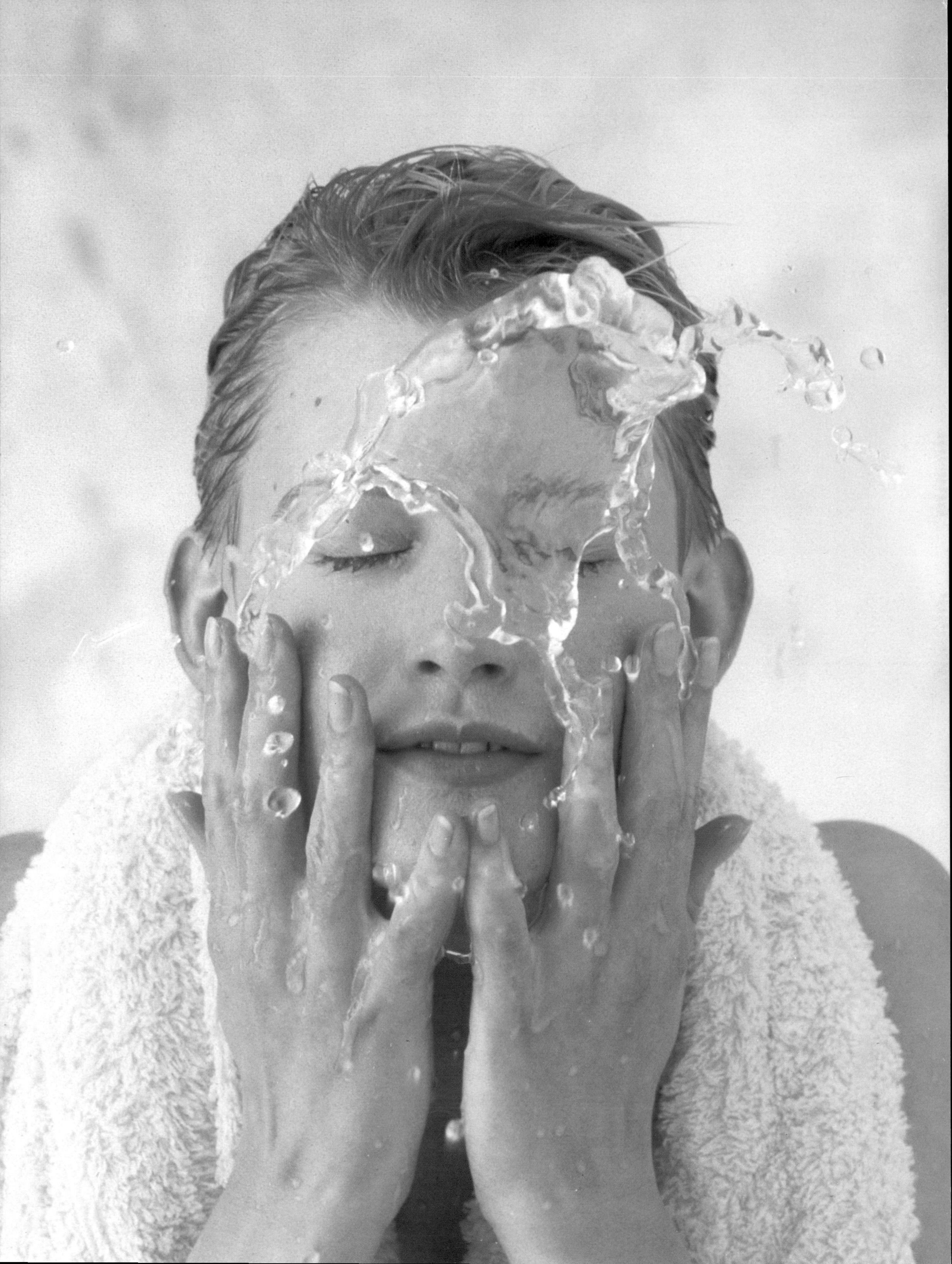

DRY SKIN

Dry skin tends to feel tight, particularly after washing with water. You feel the need for moisturizer, and your skin only feels comfortable when it is properly lubricated. Fair skin is usually dry – 85 per cent of women with light colouring have dry skin.

Dry skin is partly due to insufficient quantities of skin oil being produced, which means that water is more easily lost from the surface of the skin. But other factors also influence the dryness of the skin: air conditioning, central heating, sun and wind all have a dehydrating effect, and as skin ages so it tends to dry out. Generally more fragile than oily skin, dry skin can look thinner. Because the pores are less noticeable, the texture is finer. Be very careful not to 'drag' your skin when applying creams or make-up.

Sebum, the oil produced to lubricate the skin, has a protective action. Since dry skin has less sebum than normal skin, it is more vulnerable to the elements. You will find that you burn more easily so you have to be especially careful in the sun. Take care not to expose your skin to extreme temperatures. They can cause red veins to appear, especially on your cheeks. However, the beauty of dry skin is that it is usually free from blemishes and, if kept well-lubricated, has a wonderfully fresh and clear bloom.

All the products you use should be mild, and if you particularly like the effect of toners, make sure they contain no alcohol, which is too harsh and drying for your skin. You will need to use lashings of moisturizer – some women even find that they need it in the middle of the day as well as in the morning and at night. Of course, if you do so, it means that you have to take off your make-up first.

If you work in a well-heated or air-conditioned environment, you should investigate the use of humidifiers, which can put moisture back in to dried-out air.

To keep dry skin looking its best and feeling smooth, the topmost layer of dead skin should be gently removed with an exfoliating substance such as a special facial cleansing bar, or washing grains. Once a week should be enough, and you should use a rich moisturizer immediately afterwards. When choosing commercial face masks, go for the ones that are specifically designed for dry skin rather than the ones that harden on the face.

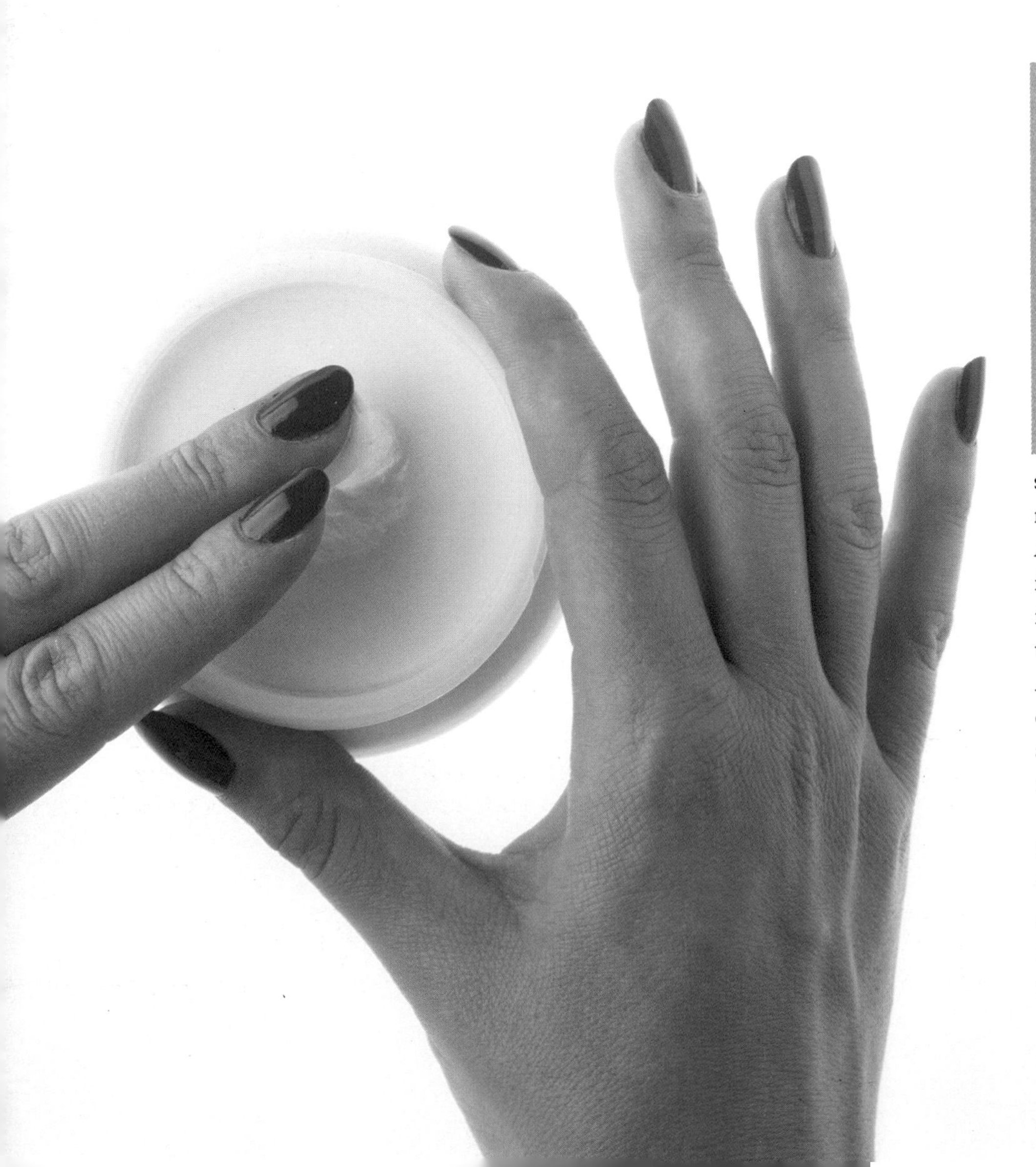

Home remedies

You should give yourself a face mask once a week, so long as the ingredients you choose condition and moisturize your skin rather than tighten and dry it. Masks that are suitable for dry skin can be used to good effect on other parts of your body as well as your face: your hands and throat, for instance.

A banana mashed with 15 ml (1 tbsp) of honey makes a moisturizing mask, which you should leave on for 20 minutes before removing. Honey on its own is also good. Avocado is an oily fruit, which means that it is also moisturizing – you can purée the flesh and pat it on your face, or simply rub the empty avocado skin over your face. Another quick mask is made by beating an egg yolk with a few drops of cider vinegar and 5 ml (1 tsp) of olive oil, and painting it on your skin with a facial brush.

A good all-over moisturizing treatment for the body involves adding either 568 ml (1 pt) of ordinary milk or 45 ml (3 tbsp) of dried milk granules to your bath water. A few drops of almond oil will make it even richer and more luxurious.

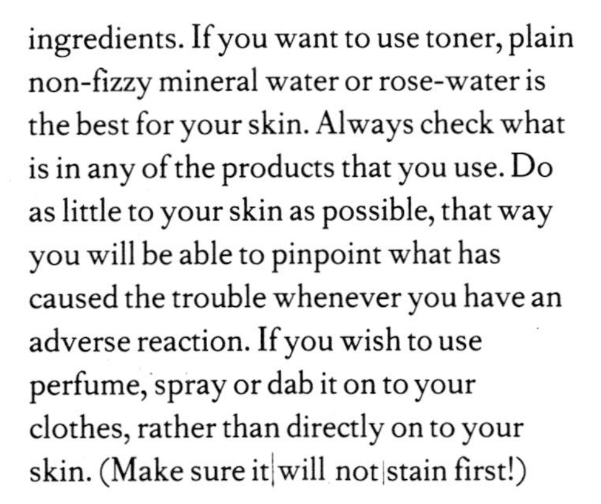

Sensitive skin is skin that reacts badly to products that you use on your skin or to foods that you eat. You may break out into spots, or your skin may puff up or redden. Some sensitive skins just react quickly to the sun or rough textures – even to wool. Any of the skin types can also be sensitive, or have sensitive areas, though it is more common to people with dry skin. The skin is an organ – the largest in the body – and it can react like any other organ to something that doesn't agree with the body.

If you have sensitive skin you will be aware to a certain extent what affects it in your case. It could be a reaction to strong foods, such as curries, which make the skin redden. It might be a more severe allergy to certain ingredients in skin creams or cosmetics, which make the skin round your eyes puff and swell. You can only be sure what is the trigger in your own case by taking care each time to note down everything you ate or used directly before you experienced an adverse reaction.

If you can find no particular pattern, it could be that the detergents or water softeners you are using to wash your clothes are to blame. A clue to this is if you notice an inflamed reaction at places where clothes – such as waistbands or bra straps – fit closely and rub.

There are hypo-allergenic products formulated for sensitive skins. The name means that they contain fewer known irritants than ordinary cosmetics, such as strong perfumes. There is, however, no totally *non*-allergenic product made and you could be sensitive to an ingredient even in these carefully prepared cosmetics. You can often find acceptable products amongst those that don't contain the hypo-allergenic label; look out for the most simple of products: unperfumed creams, soaps, and cosmetics. Shun products with long lists of ingredients and go for the ones that contain fewer and more natural ingredients. If you want to use toner, plain non-fizzy mineral water or rose-water is the best for your skin. Always check what is in any of the products that you use. Do as little to your skin as possible, that way you will be able to pinpoint what has caused the trouble whenever you have an adverse reaction. If you wish to use perfume, spray or dab it on to your clothes, rather than directly on to your skin. (Make sure it will not stain first!)

Home remedies

With sensitive skin, you might be tempted to forego any kind of regular exfoliation. But your skin also needs the occasional clearing away of dead cells. You should only use natural methods: your usual unperfumed soap on a clean face flannel, or gentle face cleansing grains on a clean, boiled face flannel, rubbed very gently into your skin. Alternatively, you can make yourself an almond-meal cleansing pack. Mix three 15 ml spoons (3 tbsp) of meal with warm water to make a thin paste, and smooth it over your face. Leave for five minutes and then wash it off with lukewarm water. Pat dry with a clean soft towel.

If you can't find a moisturizer that does not produce an allergic reaction you could use a little almond oil which has no additives. It won't feel as nice as moisturizer, but it will lubricate your skin.

For a nourishing face mask, combine one 15 ml spoon (1 tbsp) of almond meal with 15 ml (1 tbsp) of honey and an egg yolk. Mix well to achieve an even, smooth consistency and apply all over the face, excluding the eye area. Leave for 20 minutes, using the time to relax, and then wash off thoroughly by splashing with lukewarm water. Pat dry with a soft towel.

OILY SKIN

You'll know that your skin is oily simply by the look and feel of it. First thing in the morning, in strong daylight, you'll notice that it has a sheen on the surface. As the day goes on, it may begin to feel 'sticky' to the touch.

This is because it produces more than normal quantities of skin oil, which is called sebum. Another sign of this type of skin is visible 'open' pores – the openings of the sebaceous glands which produce the oil.

Oily skin is not the opposite of dry skin. They are two entirely different conditions. Skin is made oily by excess sebum. It is not only a shortage of sebum that causes a dry skin, but also a shortage of moisture. Your skin can be dry and oily at the same time. If you are trying to dry out spots by using a strong astringent all over your face, the skin in between the spots can become dry, thickened and scaly. Usually, however, the extra oil protects the skin from moisture loss.

Oily skin can be a problem for girls and young women. Because oil attracts dirt and dust, pores can quickly become blocked. As a result, blackheads and spots are formed. But there are advantages to oily skin too: its well-lubricated surface doesn't wrinkle easily. As you grow older less oil is produced, your skin 'balances' out, and so looks young longer. You can take sunbathing more readily – in fact it is often beneficial to oily skin, helping to dry up spots, for example. *But* you must use a suitable protection product – your skin can still burn.

Keep your skin scrupulously clean: use a cleansing milk to remove make-up and wash with an unperfumed soap. You could also use a wash-off cleanser if you prefer. Don't use anything too harsh to remove the oil – the glands will only work harder to replace it, making the skin surface over-dry and tough in consequence. A crucial part of the cleansing routine which you should observe is to remove the very top surface of the skin – a process known as exfoliation, which will be a great help in preventing the blockages that lead to spots and blackheads. Do it as often as you think you need to – every day if you wish – with something like oatmeal washing grains, not all over your face, but concentrating on the problem areas, around nose and chin, for instance. Use a light moisturizer after washing or exfoliating; it is moisture, not oil, which gives skin a beautiful glow. You can buy oil-free moisturizers for your kind of skin.

If you have spots or blackheads, wash your face with warm water and disinfect the blemishes with an antiseptic lotion on the tip of a cotton bud. I don't recommend squeezing them, for fear of scarring, but if you do try to remove one or two, wrap your fingers in clean tissue and press *gently* on either side. *Never* dig or press too hard.

Home remedies

Slices of cucumber, wiped gently over the face after cleansing, will tone your skin naturally; so will slices of raw potato. If you prefer to use a liquid toner on damp cotton wool, then 5 ml (1 tsp) of cider vinegar mixed into a glass of fresh water works well.

A regular face mask, once or twice a week, is very good for oily skin. The following should be left on for 20 minutes then rinsed off with warm water. Do not put masks around the eye area.

Peeled and cored ripe pears can be put in the blender or mashed, and then spread on your face – preferably over thin gauze, which holds the mask against the skin. This has a mild astringent effect.

Beaten egg white, mixed with 2.5 ml (½ tsp) of lemon juice, is quick to make.

For a mud-type mask, mix Fuller's earth with water to make a thin paste.

Black, as a definition of skin colour, is even more misleading than 'white'. One dermatologist has identified 35 different shades of black skin – compared to 10 of white skin. The colour of black skin varies from a pale caramel to deep ebony, and many dark-skinned people have a number of different tones on their face – up to four. Your forehead is usually the lightest part, the skin around your eyes the darkest.

The degree of colour in any skin depends on the amount of melanin in it. The more you have the darker your skin will be. Melanin is the body's own sunscreen – it filters the harmful rays of sunlight so that they cannot penetrate deeply enough to damage the area where new skin is made. For this reason black skins don't usually suffer the ageing effects of sunlight to the degree that white skins do, although you can burn in strong sunlight as easily if left unprotected. In general, the darker the skin the longer it will retain its youthful good looks. Even so, dark skins can, and do, tan – but it takes longer to happen.

Black skin is usually oily – often to a greater degree than oily white skin, for it has more sebaceous glands. But it can still dry out if not properly looked after, and a sign of this is a greyish, flaky look to the surface of the skin. Black skin, like white skin, can also be a combination of oily and dry areas.

Black skin should usually be treated in the same way as any other oily skin, with care taken to treat dry areas gently. Even though you are less likely to suffer from bad acne, if you have black skin, blackheads can be a problem. Against darker skin they are harder to see, so you should be particularly scrupulous about cleansing the areas on which they are likely to occur – around your nose and on your chin. Don't be tempted to use harsh astringents to control oiliness, because they will dull the glow of your skin by over-drying the surface. Skin bleaches are not to be recommended either. They do not affect the fundamental pigmentation of the skin because the amount of melanin you produce remains the same. The lightening effect is only temporary, therefore. What's worse is that they give a dusty, dull look to your complexion.

Home remedies

Use any of the natural remedies recommended for oily skin. On any drier areas, use the conditioning treatments for dry skin.

An effective exfoliating mask can also be made from papaya flesh, pulped and spread on to your face for 20 minutes, and then rinsed off with warm water. A mask to refine and freshen your skin when it feels tired can be made from mixing powdered skim milk with enough lemon juice mixed 50:50 with water to make a creamy paste. Again, leave it on for 20 minutes before you rinse it off. A quick and easy mask, which you can apply to the dry areas of your face at the same time, is good quality bought mayonnaise – which contains eggs, olive oil and vinegar. You can make your own, of course, either in the traditional way, or in a blender. Break a whole egg into the blender goblet and dribble olive or sunflower oil on to it while the blender is running, until a creamy consistency is formed. Finally add 15 ml (1 tbsp) of cider or wine vinegar. If you want to soothe your eyes while waiting for the mask to take effect, lie back and place thin slices of cucumber over your eyelids.

QUESTIONS & ANSWERS

Is there a beauty problem which has been troubling you for some time? Here Barbara supplies the answers to some of your most common queries.

What is the difference between fresheners, toners and astringents?

Astringent lotions are for the correction of oily skin and the closure of pores following the application of cleansing creams and lotions. In general, all contain the milder aluminium salts, some alcohol and the aromatic flower waters such as rose and orange. Skin tonics are used for cleansing and the care of facial skin, are cooling and refreshing, and are often described as skin fresheners. Preparations which come under this heading may include diluted 'astringent lotions' or freshening lotions based essentially on alcohol or eau-de-cologne with witch hazel. A little borax or other mild alkali might be included. Some skin tonics and fresheners are described as 'alcohol-free' and are usually recommended for fine or sensitive skin.

What is the difference between moisturizer and night cream?

All moisturizing creams are made in a similar way, but moisturizers which are formulated for use during the day contain oil with a high melting point, which means that they do not feel greasy, and seem to vanish when applied to the skin. Night creams are usually denser and feel greasier when first put on. They are not well-suited for use under foundations.

Are expensive skin-care products more effective?

Not necessarily. Some of the cheapest skin-care products on the market are good, as they are made with natural ingredients and not too many additives. Remember that a great deal of the cost of skin-care products goes into packaging and advertising. It's constancy in skin care that counts.

Suddenly my skin is looking and feeling awful – but I haven't changed the products I use – why is this?

Skin changes. It ages, and may go from oily, say, to rather dry, which means you would have to change your skin-care routine. You might also need different products at different times of the year. During the winter, for instance, I use a heavier moisturizing cream because my skin dries out more in a centrally heated atmosphere. A change of routine might be necessary because, apart from anything else, skin care should be interesting and fun – not just a chore.

How long can you keep skin creams?

Most commercial skin creams can be kept indefinitely because they contain preservative. If you have made the cream yourself, or the label clearly states that no preservative is used, then you should keep it in the fridge. But remember, if you discover that an otherwise perfectly fresh cream or lotion irritates your face, you may be able to use it as a body moisturizer.

Cream stays on my face for ages – how long should I leave it to sink in?

Blot with tissue to remove any excess after 20 minutes. Your skin is also a protective shield so creams don't continue sinking in – they sit on the surface, and any excess does no extra good at all, which means you don't have to leave passion-killing amounts on your face at bedtime! Massage any leftover cream into your hands and elbows.

What can I do to ensure that my skin really benefits from my moisturizer?

Warm damp skin absorbs better than cold dry skin. I find that putting moisturizer on after a bath or after just washing my face gives the best results of all. The dampness is trapped under the moisturizer – so it truly does moisturize the skin.

I have oily skin – do I really need a moisturizer?

Yes, but a light one. It is moisture in your skin that makes it supple and stay young-looking. The oil in your skin stops some of the moisture from evaporating, but it is not fully effective on its own – it needs help from a moisturizer. Avoid the central oily patches, and – after cleansing – put the moisturizer on your cheeks, forehead, throat and around your eyes.

Why must you be so careful with skin around eyes?

There are very few strong muscles and little flesh around the eyes – little more than skin covering the gap between socket and eyeball, so treat this area with extra care.

I have very dark areas under my eyes – are these eye bags, and how do I disguise them?

A dark area under the eye is a shadow – a dent. You can cover shadows successfully with concealer. Eyebags are different – they stick out above the shadow, varying from a small lip to a large bulge. You can't really conceal them with make-up. Concealer – which is lighter than foundation – simply makes them more prominent.

Can I get rid of the bags under my eyes?

If you are not ill, under the weather or suffering from too little sleep, yet your eyes tend to bag – then your bags are probably hereditary, and only plastic surgery will remove them properly. Temporary bags can be caused by illness or lack of sleep – and using too greasy a cream around the eye. If your cream is the culprit, switch to a lighter one. If over-indulgence or late nights are the causes there are a number of things you can do to reduce the swelling. People swear by different remedies: drinking a glass of hot water; using commerical eyepads, or used, cooled, tea bags, or slices of cucumber placed over the eyes. I always vow to get a good night's sleep as soon as possible.

How often should I exfoliate my skin?

Dry skin probably only needs exfoliating once a week. Oily or particularly dingy skin might need it more often – gently, once a day if you wish. Incidentally, you don't have to do your entire face each time – you can concentrate on the areas that tend to build up grime – such as round your nose or chin.

Can I use a rough face flannel for exfoliating my face?

I'm against flannels unless you are prepared to use a fresh, clean one *every day* and boil it up after use – otherwise they spread germs.

I occasionally get spots – how should I treat them when this happens?

If the spot has a head, wash your face with warm water, disinfect the spot with antiseptic lotion on a cotton bud and squeeze it very gently with fingers well wrapped in tissue. Finally, dab it with antiseptic lotion and let it be. If it doesn't clear easily, leave well alone. Never mark your skin. It is better not to wear make-up over the spots, but if you do, then try medicated foundation and concealer sticks.

Unfortunately, some people find they are allergic to the ingredients in medicated products, so watch out for adverse reactions.

If you have the kind of spots that crop up around the time of your period, which are caused by hormone activity rather than blockage in the pores, it is fine to wear make-up, and you will find that they go of their own accord. Problems will only occur if you don't clean the foundation off properly at the end of the day.

I never feel really clean unless I wash my face. But my skin is dry. Is it bad for me?

Every type of skin can be washed and it is perfectly OK – especially if you like doing it. But bear in mind a couple of points. If you use soap choose an unperfumed bar. You can use cleansing bars that look like soap but which are simply solid cleansers – and they are gentler than soap. There are also face washes and rinseable cleansers that come in liquid form, but can be rinsed off with water. Whichever you choose, rinse really well afterwards – don't leave a trace on your skin. If it is mainly the feel of water that you like, you can finish off a normal cleansing routine with a spray of still mineral water, which is commercially packaged in a spray can. I make my own by putting mineral water in a plant spray bottle.

What can I do to close open pores?

You can't change pore size. What you must do is keep skin scrupulously clean and exfoliate often, so it looks translucent and light all the time.

Astringents are not a good idea – they seem to have a temporary pore-closing effect because they slightly irritate the skin, making it swell up so that the pores look smaller. What they also do is harden the surface of the skin as they dry it out. Natural astringents, such as cucumber, are as powerful as is necessary.

Open pores can be disguised to a certain degree by make-up – face powder is good, as it fills them in. Again, cleanse off thoroughly at the end of the day.

Are regular facials necessary?

There's no doubt about it – yes. Masks clean the skin thoroughly and steaming is beneficial as it makes the skin soft, warm and receptive to cream. Have one once a month – the 30 minutes' or so relaxation involved is good for you too.

Because I have pale eyelashes, I look very washed-out without mascara – for example, first thing in the morning or when I am on a beach holiday. Can you suggest a solution?

The easy and effective answer is to dye your eyelashes very dark brown or black, depending on your skin tone. You can do this yourself with one of the proprietary preparations available. Full instructions for use are given and you should follow these very carefully. An alternative is to have them dyed in a beauty salon, perhaps as the last step in a professional facial as part of the treatment or as a separate process. The effects last as long as it takes for your lashes to renew themselves – generally about four to six weeks, or long enough to last for a summer holiday.

Can face masks improve sallow skin colour?

When I'm pale in the summer I crush up strawberries and spread them over my face on top of a piece of gauze, which stops the pulp sliding off. After ten minutes I rinse it off, and then add plenty of moisturizer. The strawberries are slightly astringent, and also give a pleasant pink tinge to the skin.

Which other home remedies do you recommend?

My favourites are avocados: I sometimes rub the skin over my face after I've eaten one, or I rub it into my elbows – it is extremely moisturizing. Crushed papaya used as a mask is healing. You can make other good masks by mixing natural ingredients into skin cream: egg, oatmeal, or olive oil. After squeezing the juice, I use the lemon halves to take stains off my hands – but it is astringent so I rub something lubricating into my hands afterwards. Lemon juice is also a natural hair bleacher when combed through before sitting in the sun.

What can I do about my double chin?

Double chins are caused by excess fat, in which case dieting is the only answer; or bad posture, so that learning to stand and sit up straight helps to minimize the double chin; or else it is simply the structure of your face, in which case you can't do very much to help it. Unfortunately, this is one of the things you can't conceal with make-up, though choice of neckline can disguise the problem.

Can any cream get rid of my wrinkles?

Unfortunately not, but you can slow down the process of wrinkling, and to some extent stop the wrinkles getting worse. Ultraviolet is the main culprit: all daylight, and particularly strong sunlight, will age your skin fast and predispose it to wrinkling, one reason why unlimited sunbathing is not a good thing. Use a foundation with ultraviolet protection – specifically advertised as a sun-block base. Alternatively, put sun block on every morning, winter and summer, mixed with your moisturizer, or, as I do in summer, use it as a moisturizer all by itself. The parts of your face that age first: eyes, neck and round the mouth, should be treated with care. Don't pull or stretch the skin round your eyes, or it will sag and wrinkle; moisturize your neck at the same time as the rest of your face; and remember that smoking will not only create pucker wrinkles around your mouth, but because tobacco takes Vitamin C out of your system it also accelerates the wrinkling process.

How can I avoid developing liver spots on my hands?

Unfortunately, liver spots do generally appear with age, but you can retard their appearance by using the same sun block as you use for your face on your hands as well.

I tend to have a high colour, and thread veins on my cheeks and nose — what should I do about this?

Extremes of temperature make veins contract and expand, and sometimes the tiny veins rupture.

Protect your face well at all times and avoid too much steam and heat. Green make-up will disguise high colour, but always put it on very carefully by a window in good natural light, — I'd rather see over-pink cheeks than green ones!

I am so embarrassed about my facial hair. What can I do about it?

If it is just a light moustache, but dark in colour, then you can use facial bleach to fade it until it is barely noticeable.

However, if it is a dark brown all over, or you have a lot of hair, then it should be treated by a professional beautician who will advise you whether you need to have it removed by electrolysis, or by hot wax.

If you only have a few stray long hairs you can use facial depilatory cream, facial wax, or pluck them out with tweezers. There is no truth that plucking is at all harmful, so long as you obey the basic rules. Your skin, hands and tweezers must be clean. You should grasp the hair firmly at the root and always pull in the direction the hair is growing.

If I remove the hair on my face will it grow back heavier and darker?

It is a fallacy that hair grows back heavier, stronger or darker afterwards. Only a hair similar to the one that was there before can grow from each follicle, and the colour it grows will always be the same. In fact, quite the reverse is true; constant removal — especially by plucking or waxing — eventually weakens the hair in the follicle.

Why is it inadvisable to cut or shave unwanted hair?

This is because the hair grows back with its cut-off end blunt and the re-growth has the bristly feel of men's beards. Removed in other ways the hair grows back with its normal pointed end, which makes it feel silky.

Do you advise shaving *any* unwanted hair?

I think that shaving the hair under the arms is all right, because it is so quickly and easily done that you are unlikely to let yourself get to the prickly stage.

I wanted to wax the 'bikini line' hairs along with my legs, but friends have said it is harmful — is this so?

Not at all. I have bikini line and half-leg waxing done regularly, which keeps it in control.

How often should I moisturize body skin?

Every day, preferably after a bath or shower when your skin is warm and damp. You don't need expensive creams to do this. I keep a dispenser bottle filled with odds and ends of cream and oil — remnants of hand cream and body oil — by the bath to use. If you use an ordinary cheap-and-cheerful body cream, mixing it with a bit of almond oil enrichens it. If you have an oily back you don't have to put cream on it every time you do the rest of your body. Cocoa butter, which is cheap, is excellent for dry areas of the body. Some of my friends swear that, mixed with Vitamin E oil, it also helps prevent the marks caused by the skin stretching because of changes in weight.

It is particularly important not to neglect moisturizing your body when you are exposing a lot of it to the sun. This means not only during, but also before and after sunbathing.

Does the body need exfoliating too?

Yes. You can see for yourself on a beach holiday: your skin is better, softer, silkier than usual. That's because of natural exfoliation: the top layer of body skin is constantly being rubbed by sand and salt sea water, and lots of oil is then smoothed in while the skin is warm and receptive. A good trick at home is to scrub yourself down with a handful of sea salt once a week after you have finished your bath. Then rinse off well and moisturize plentifully afterwards. Concentrate particularly on the areas that get dry or spotty, like elbows, backs of arms, your bottom. You can also use oatmeal for rough patches, or salt mixed with cream. A loofah or washing mitt is also good for giving your skin a special, invigorating bathtime treat.

Do you think that body massage has any lasting benefits?

It depends what you expect it to do for you. Even on a frequent, regular basis it will not help you lose weight (although the masseuse will probably burn up a few calories!) But it does have some real advantages: the most obvious is that it is pleasant and relaxing, and if you are relaxed your muscles function better. Combined with improving the circulation, the result is glowing skin — and your skin will be softer too, if the massage is done with moisturizing oils.

EYEBROWS

Your eyebrows add shape to your face and frame your eyes. Luckily, the fashion now is for natural brows – only a little tidying up of your own shape, thickness and colour. That makes it easy to follow the best rule: to pluck only in order to enhance what you have naturally.

A very thin plucked line is ageing, and won't balance your features. It also dates you – the last time it was fashionable was at least ten years ago. You can't make naturally thin eyebrows look bushy, though you can give them a slightly thicker look by drawing in fine pencil lines (see make-up tips on page 46).

Heavily pencilled brows are also dating – which is only all right if you are trying consciously for a 'fifties look.

Eyebrows affect your expression – especially round the bridge of the nose – pluck them too wide and they will give you a vacant, or startled expression; allow them to meet in the centre and they make you look angry or disgruntled.

Eyebrows look best if they grow flat. You can encourage them to do so by smoothing petroleum jelly on to them with your fingers. Another trick is to spray lacquer on to an old toothbrush and brush them flat. Long bushy eyebrows can be trimmed slightly – and very carefully – with nail scissors.

PLUCKING

You can't go wrong if you simply clean up the natural shape of your eyebrow, without trying any elaborate reshaping. The line should not be too thin for your face, and you should not try to thin the brow out by plucking in the centre, or you'll end up with bare and uneven patches.

You can pluck above the line of the brow as well, if you don't like the shape or feel it looks wrong. This may be the case if you have a low forehead and very dark hair.

1 Assemble your equipment: **headband** to keep the hair off your face while you pluck; **pencil/ tailcomb/ long-handled cosmetic brush** for assessing where your eyebrow should start at the bridge of the nose; **good pair of chisel-ended tweezers** – the best shape for gripping the hair; **mild antiseptic and cotton wool** to swab the eyebrow area before you begin plucking, and again when you have finished.

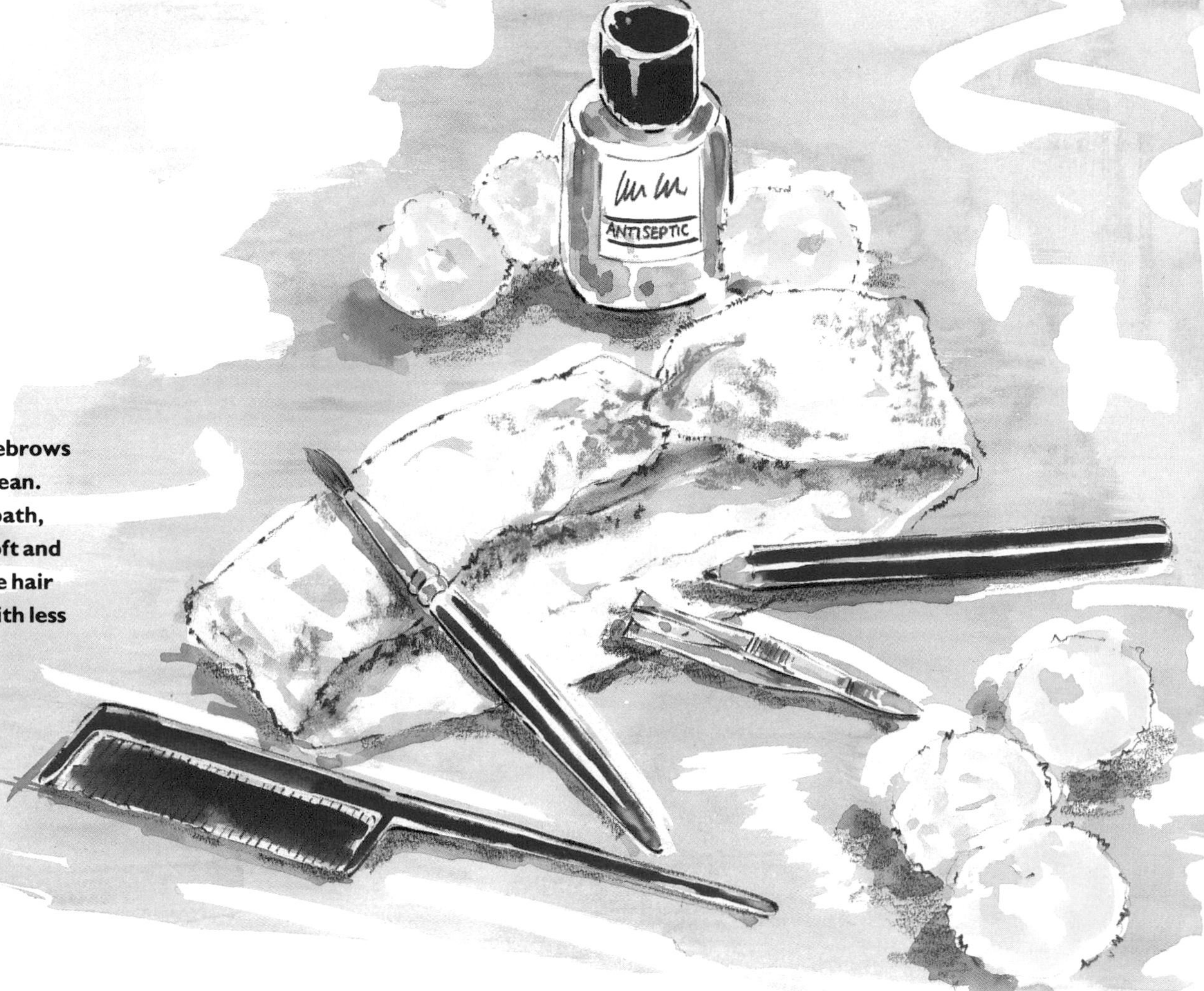

Only pluck your eyebrows when your face is clean. After, or during, a bath, when your skin is soft and warm is ideal, as the hair can be pulled out with less tugging.

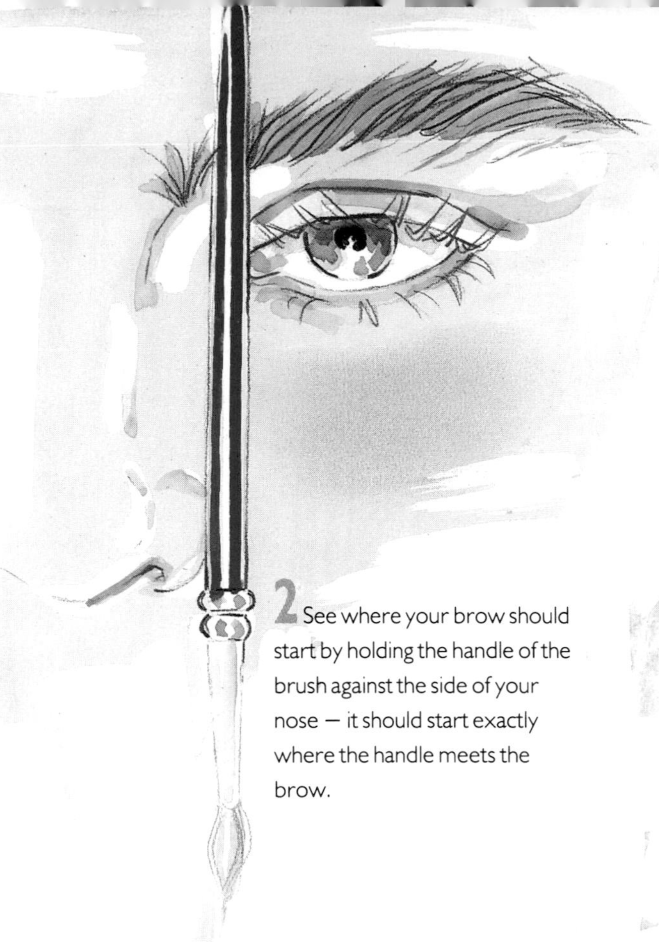

3 Stretch the skin of the eye area taut between the first two fingers on your hand.

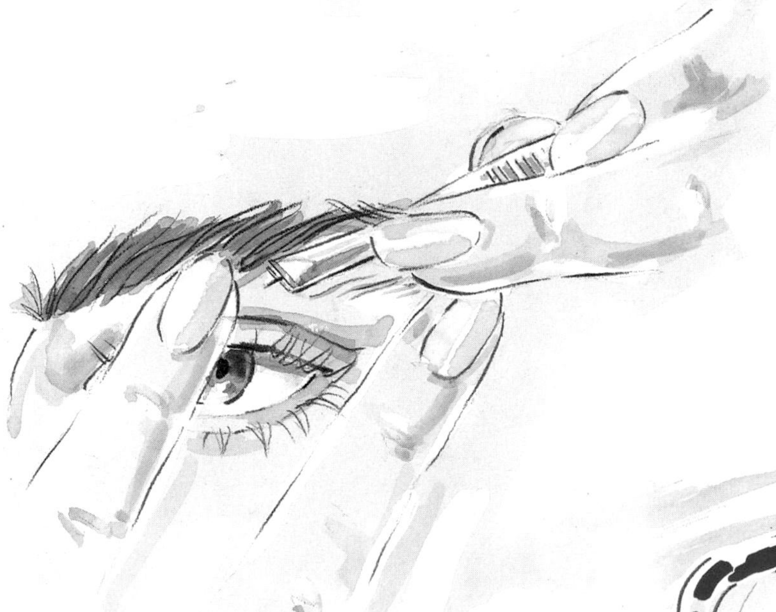

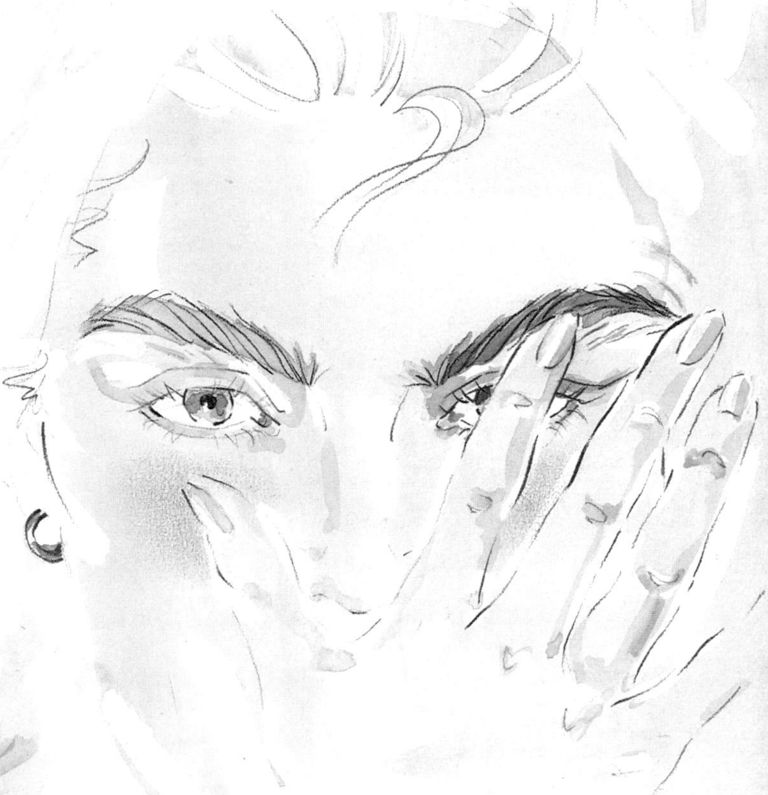

2 See where your brow should start by holding the handle of the brush against the side of your nose — it should start exactly where the handle meets the brow.

5 Pluck the stragglers first, then check the line of both eyebrows together in the mirror. Pluck so that the line of the under-curve is smooth, not wiggly or shaped like a comma.

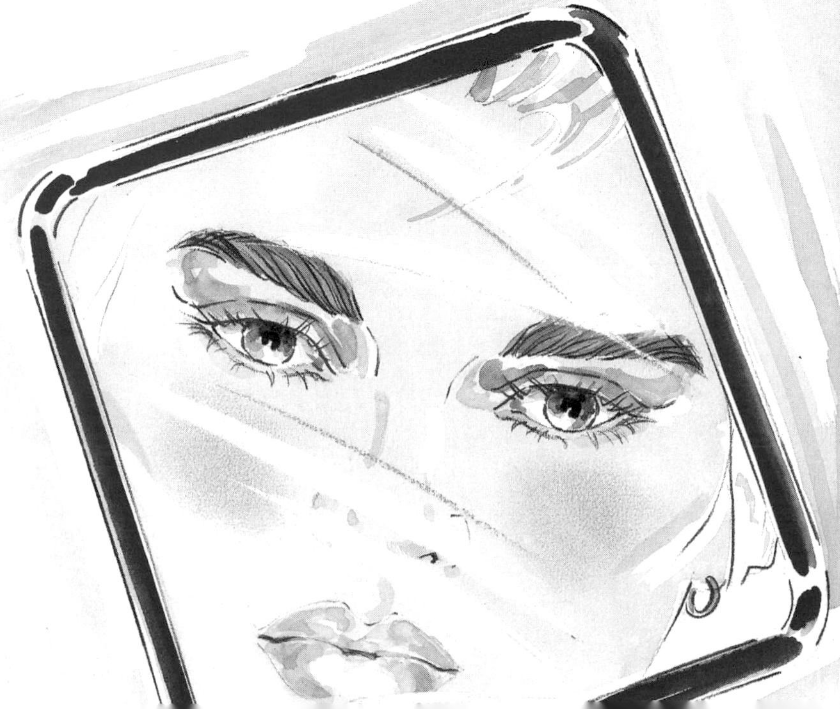

4 Place the flat end of the tweezers against your skin, and grip the hair near the root. Pull in the direction it is growing. Plucking in the wrong direction damages the follicle and causes the hair to grow crooked. Pull smoothly so as not to snap the hair off.

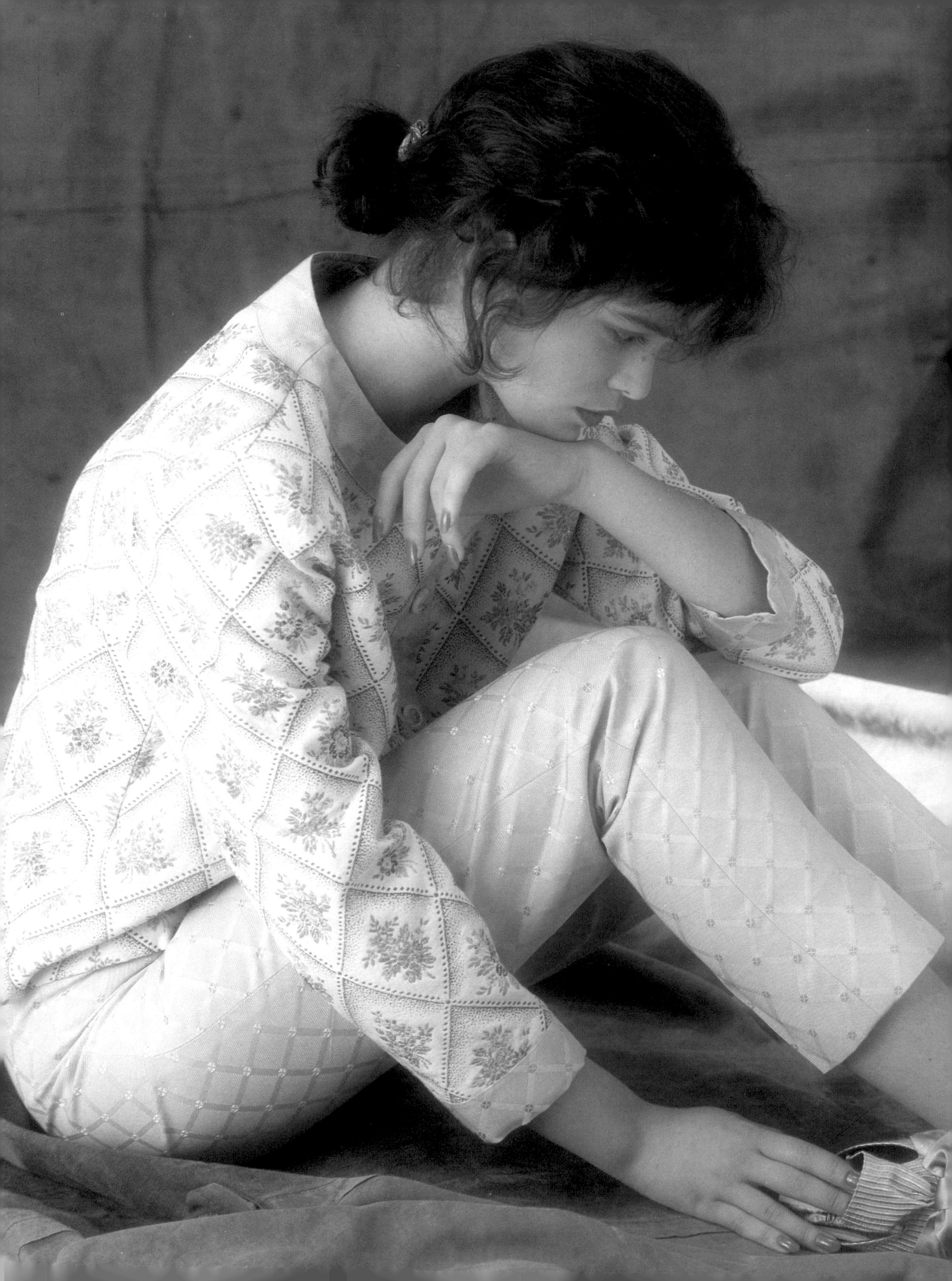

HANDS & FEET

Your hands come in for a lot of rough treatment – like your face they are continually exposed, but unlike your face they are dunked in harsh detergents and used for all manner of dirty jobs. The problem is also that hands are not very fleshy so the skin on them ages fast – like the area around your eyes – unless it is given constant care and protection. Feet need attention too: crammed into shoes and expected to carry you for miles, when it comes to body care they are quite often sadly neglected. You may find you only think of them when they are to be seen in public: on a beach holiday, or when you slip into sandals. But if they are going to look good when you need them to, it is necessary to take care of them all year round.

If you have any problems with your feet, go to a chiropodist regularly. This is particularly necessary if you have hard skin, as trying to remove it yourself can be unsatisfactory and dangerous.

Exercising every day can help you not to become stiff and arthritic later. A couple of minutes of simple exercises while you lie in bed before getting up can help loosen your hands and feet. Make your hands into fists, and then fling out your fingers two or three times. Then rotate your wrists and give your hands a good shake. For your feet, rotate your ankles and then wiggle your toes. Spread your toes as wide apart as you can.

Jacket & Trousers: Crolla · Shoes: Manolo Blahnik·

Protect your hands at all times. Get into the habit of rubbing in some hand cream every time you have had to put them in water. Wear gloves appropriate to every job you do: rubber gloves when you wash up; cotton for housework; gardening gloves when you are weeding – and of course ordinary gloves when you are outside in the cold.

If your hands are persistently dry, you can occasionally try a trick of mine: work in a mixture of olive or almond oil and cream at night and put on some white cotton gloves to hold it next to the skin while it sinks in. When putting on body lotions, remember to rub the excess cream into your feet.

A good habit to get into while you are taking a bath, and your skin is soft and warm, is to push the cuticles on your toes back gently with your thumb.

NAIL PROBLEMS

White spots are generally caused by damage to the nail bed or by mild calcium deficiency, and they can be covered with polish. Flaking, brittle nails should be kept short and cared for with cuticle cream and a nail hardener. This can be the sign of a poor diet. Check that you are eating enough vegetables, fruit and dairy products.

When your nails are very bad, you can have acrylic nails stuck over your own. Both application and removal must be done professionally at a salon; if you try to remove them yourself you risk damaging the nail underneath.

MANICURE

Give yourself a full manicure once a week. Meanwhile, if your nail varnish chips slightly, simply retouch – too much nail polish remover is not good for your nails. A split nail can be patched with a small piece of tissue covered with clear polish. Always carry an emery board with you so that you can smooth away a chip in the nail before it becomes a break.

Manicure kit

A small bowl, nail polish remover, a towel, hand cream, an emery board, an orange stick, cuticle cream, cuticle clipper, cotton wool, a nailbrush, nail care cream, base coat, nail polish and top coat. For feet: spacers for toes, large bowl, pumice stick, lotion, nail scissors.

The stages of treatment are similar for hands and feet. When doing both start with your feet.

1 Remove all old varnish **2** Simply cut toe nails straight across with scissors **3** Shape fingernails with an emery board, filing in one stroke from the side to the centre **4** Rub nail cream all around cuticles **5** Soak your nails in warm soapy water briefly to soften cuticles and hangnails **6** Scrub your nails with a nail brush. Remove stubborn dirt with the orange stick. Dry your hands **7** Rub hard skin on feet with a pumice stone **8** Rub hand cream or lotion into hands and feet **9** Apply cuticle remover. Push back cuticles with the hoof end of the orange stick, then wash the remover away. **10** Remove hang nails and excess skin with cuticle clipper. Do not clip away too much **11** If you don't plan to wear polish for a while, massage in some nail care cream. Otherwise, you're ready for . . .

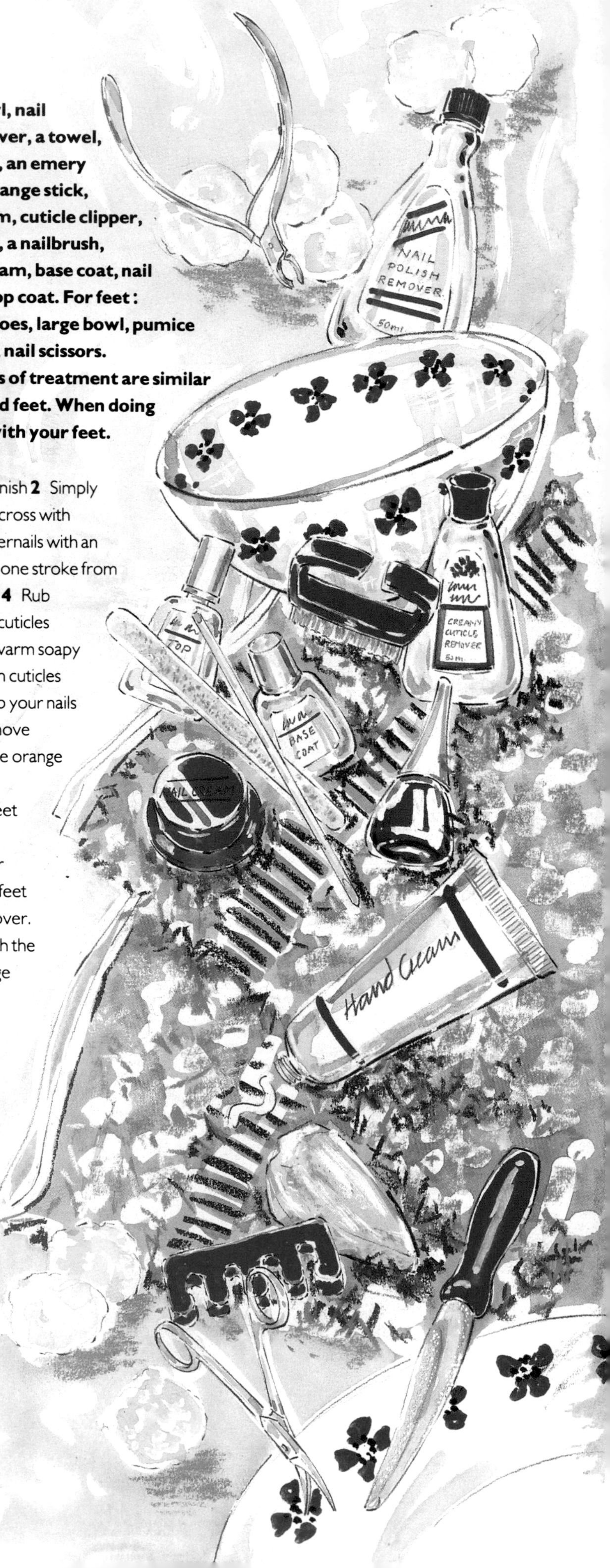

THE PERFECT PAINT JOB

Before starting, check that your nails are smooth and unridged. If they need it, apply ridge-filler first and wait for it to dry before putting on any varnish. Grip your elbows to your sides to steady your hands as you work. Put spacers between your toes to keep them separate.

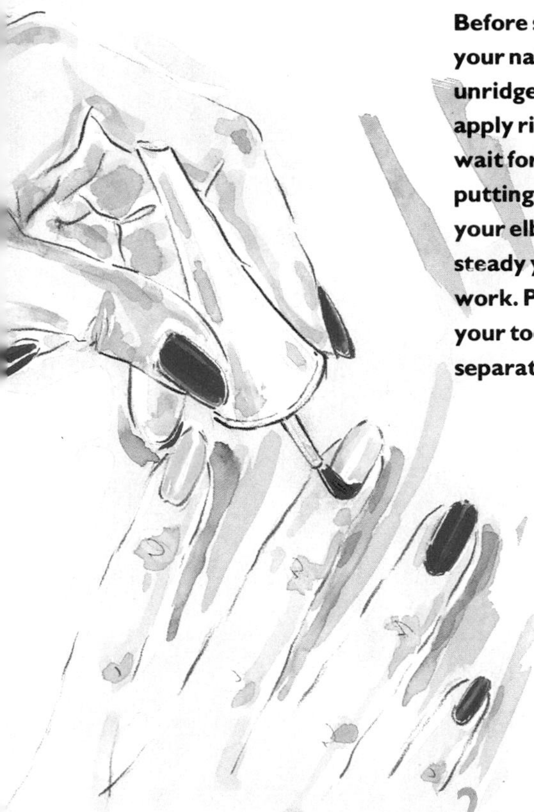

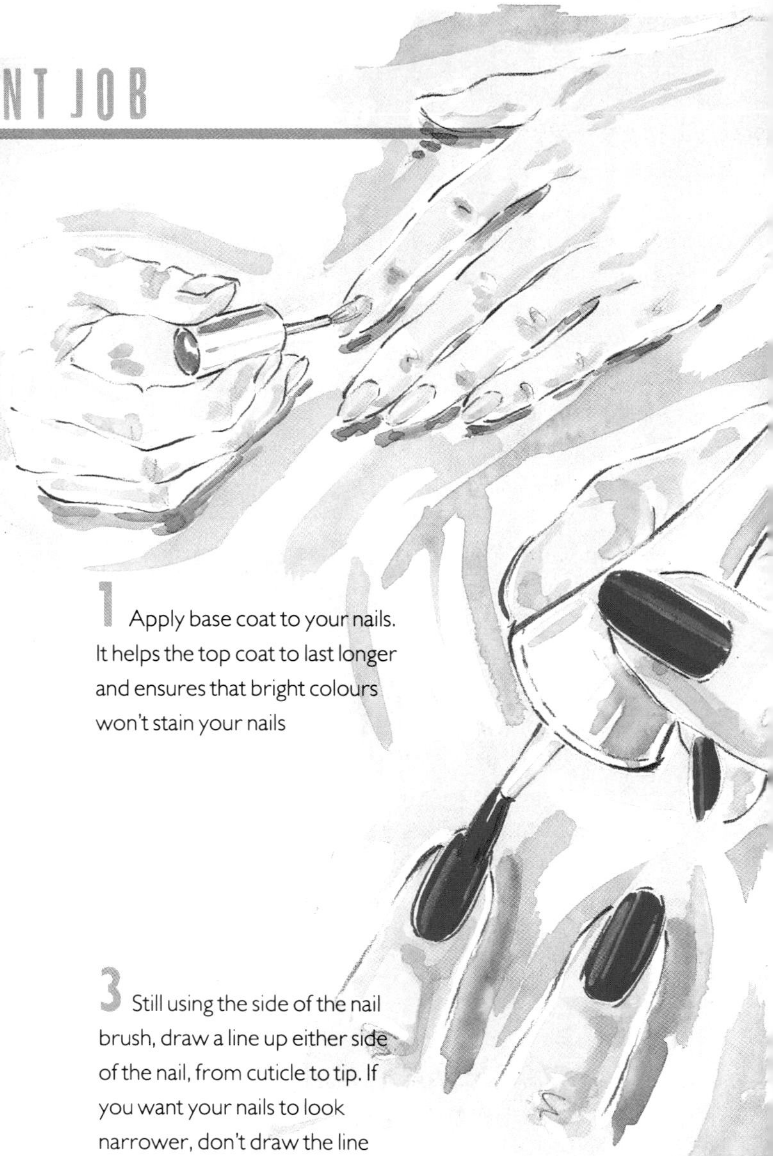

1 Apply base coat to your nails. It helps the top coat to last longer and ensures that bright colours won't stain your nails

2 Starting with your little finger, draw a loop of varnish around the line of cuticle, using the side of the nail varnish brush

3 Still using the side of the nail brush, draw a line up either side of the nail, from cuticle to tip. If you want your nails to look narrower, don't draw the line right at the edge of the nail

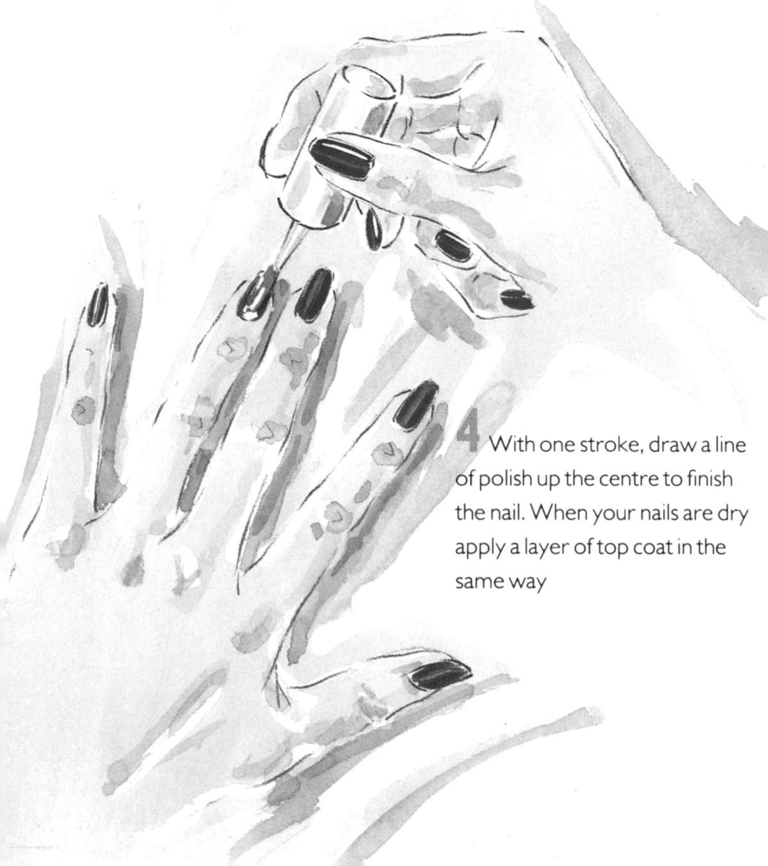

4 With one stroke, draw a line of polish up the centre to finish the nail. When your nails are dry apply a layer of top coat in the same way

If you don't want to use nail polish, you can buff your nails instead. Using nail buffing cream and a buffer, polish your nails across – first in one direction, then in the other.

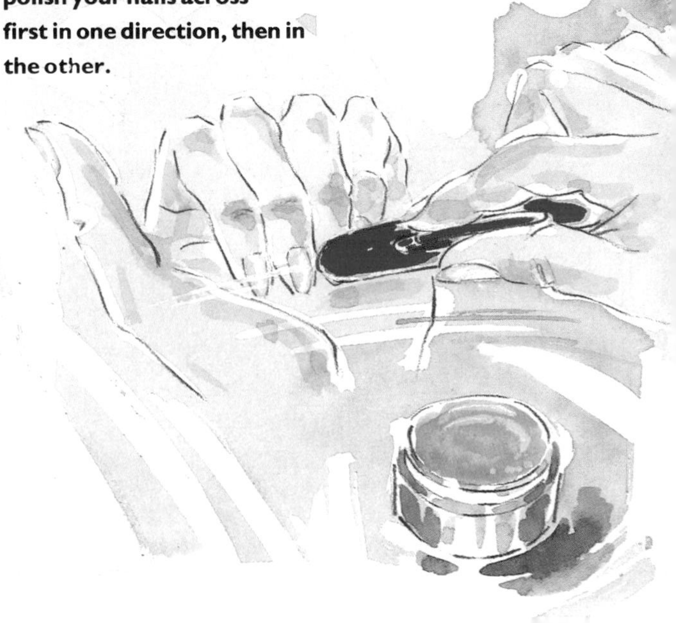

HAIR

Good looking, well-cut hair is your most important accessory and says as much about you as the clothes you wear. You can change your look quite dramatically by changing your hairstyle, with the comforting thought that if the new look is not a success it is not for ever — it will grow again! Almost anything you do to your hair is reversible — unlike your skin, which never fully recovers from lack of care.

Like your skin, the basic condition of your hair is a reflection of your general health at the time when it was being made. As each hair has an average life of between two and six years, even longer for Asian girls, your hair condition may be affected for a long time after an illness, say, or a period of eating poorly. But if you treat it with care you can make sure it looks at its best all the time.

You can make your hair any colour you want — pink, green, ash blonde, mahogany. But unless you are determined to do something really wild, you will get the best, most effective results from a colour only a shade or two different from your own, or your skin tone will look wrong against it. Think hard before trying an extreme shade, like raven or platinum blonde, as it rarely succeeds. There are many ways to colour your hair:

Permanent colorants

These penetrate to the core of the hair, replacing the natural pigment with the new colour. The effects of course are not truly permanent: they only last until the roots show through, as only visible hair is affected. Because you will see regrowth roots within a week it is important to choose a colour quite close to your own, or have the roots retouched regularly by an expert. Bleaching the hair lighter — by even one shade — is also permanent.

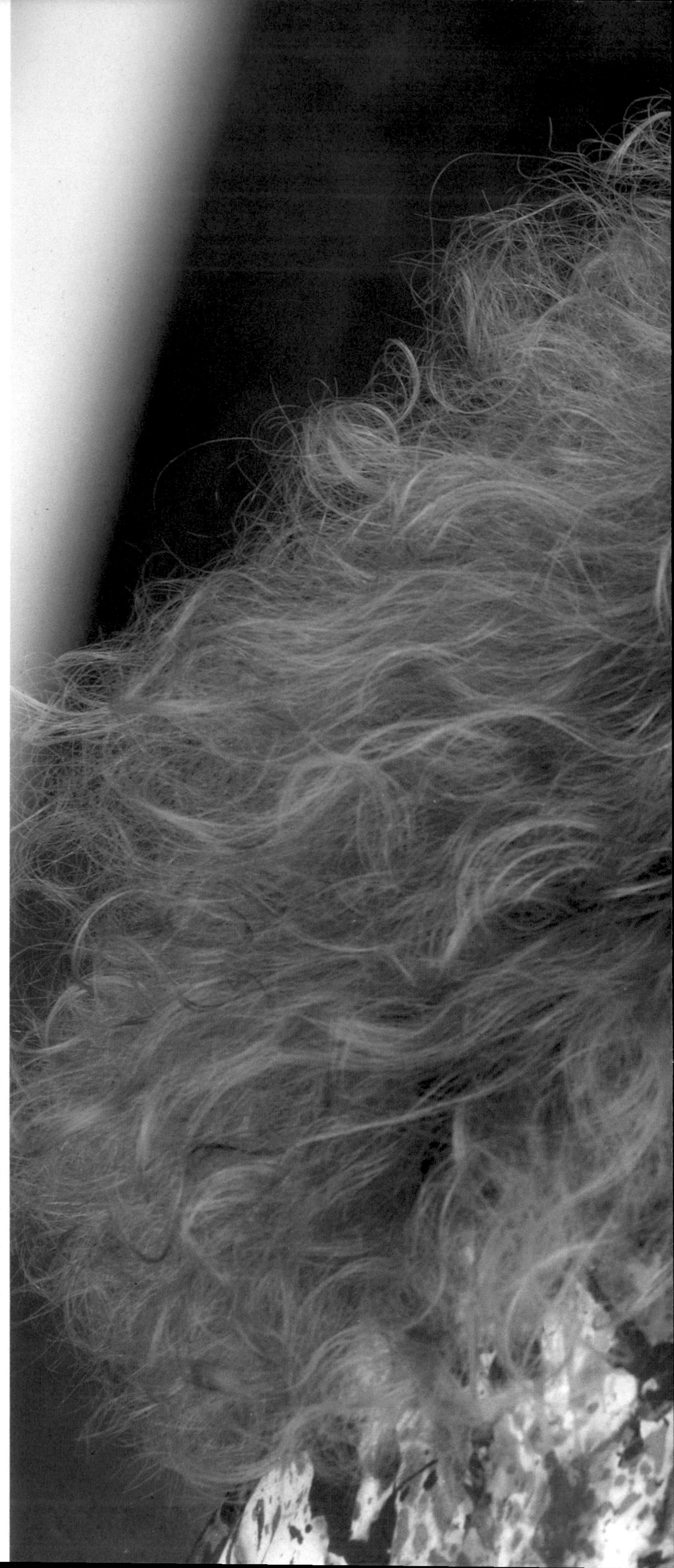

Shirt: Swanky Modes · Jewellery: Gary Wright & Sheila Teague ·

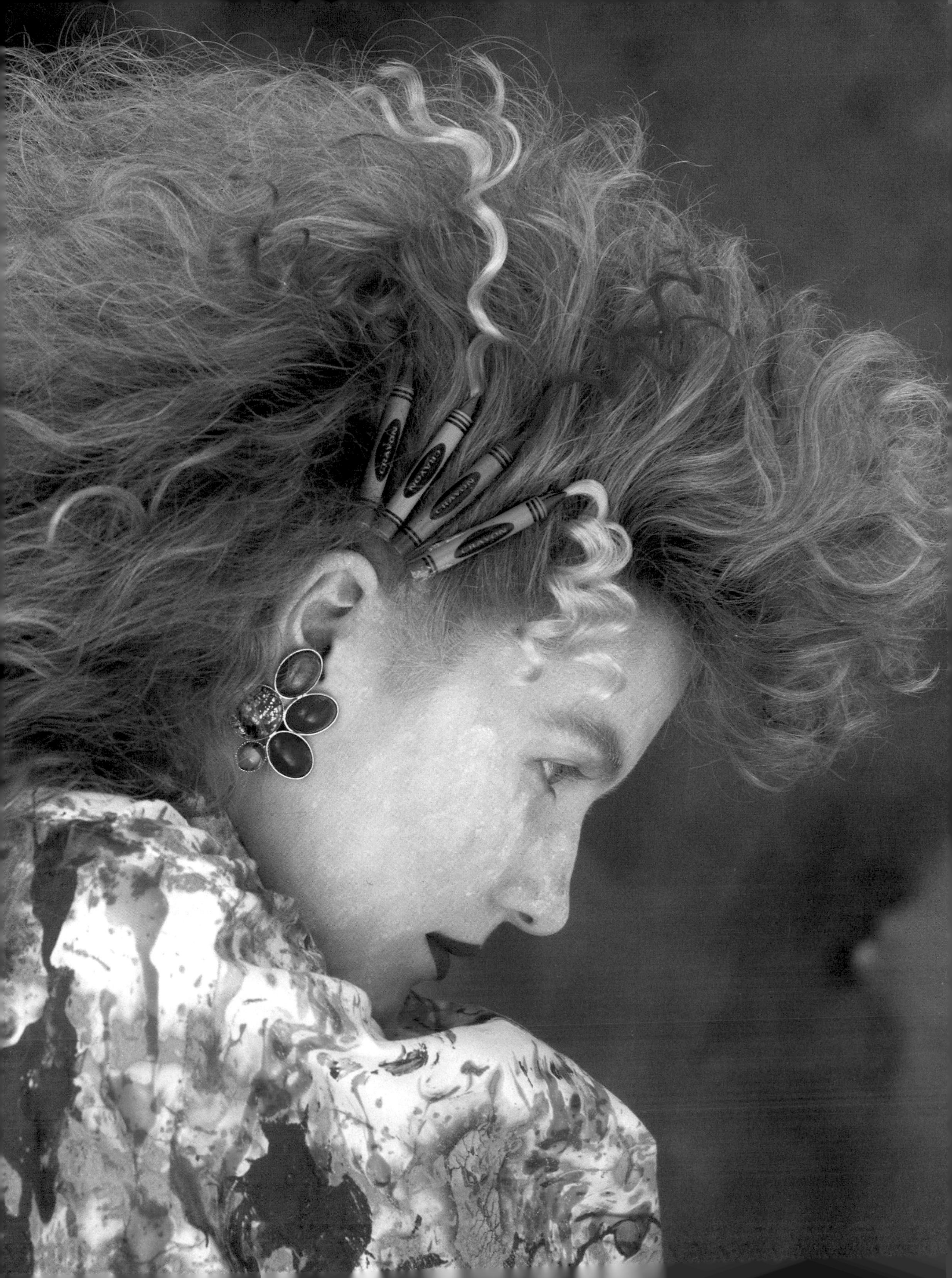
CRAYON
CRAYON
CRAYON
CRAYON

Streaks, highlights and lowlights
These may be permanent, but because only strands of the hair are affected there is not such a problem with regrowth. Your roots can be done less frequently or left to grow out altogether.
Semi-permanent colorants
These gradually wash out over a period of two to eight weeks, and usually incorporate a conditioning agent. Because the colour washes out there is no need to retouch the roots.
Temporary tints
These are wash-in rinses which wash out again at the next shampoo.
Natural colorants
Henna is a natural vegetable compound that adds rich red tones to the hair. The colour fades gradually but does not wash out. Lemon juice is a natural bleaching agent.
Make-up for hair
You can jazz up your hair just for an evening out by clipping in coloured hair strands or adding colour in the form of foams or coloured gels. Glitter also looks good in the hair – but don't let it get in your eyes.

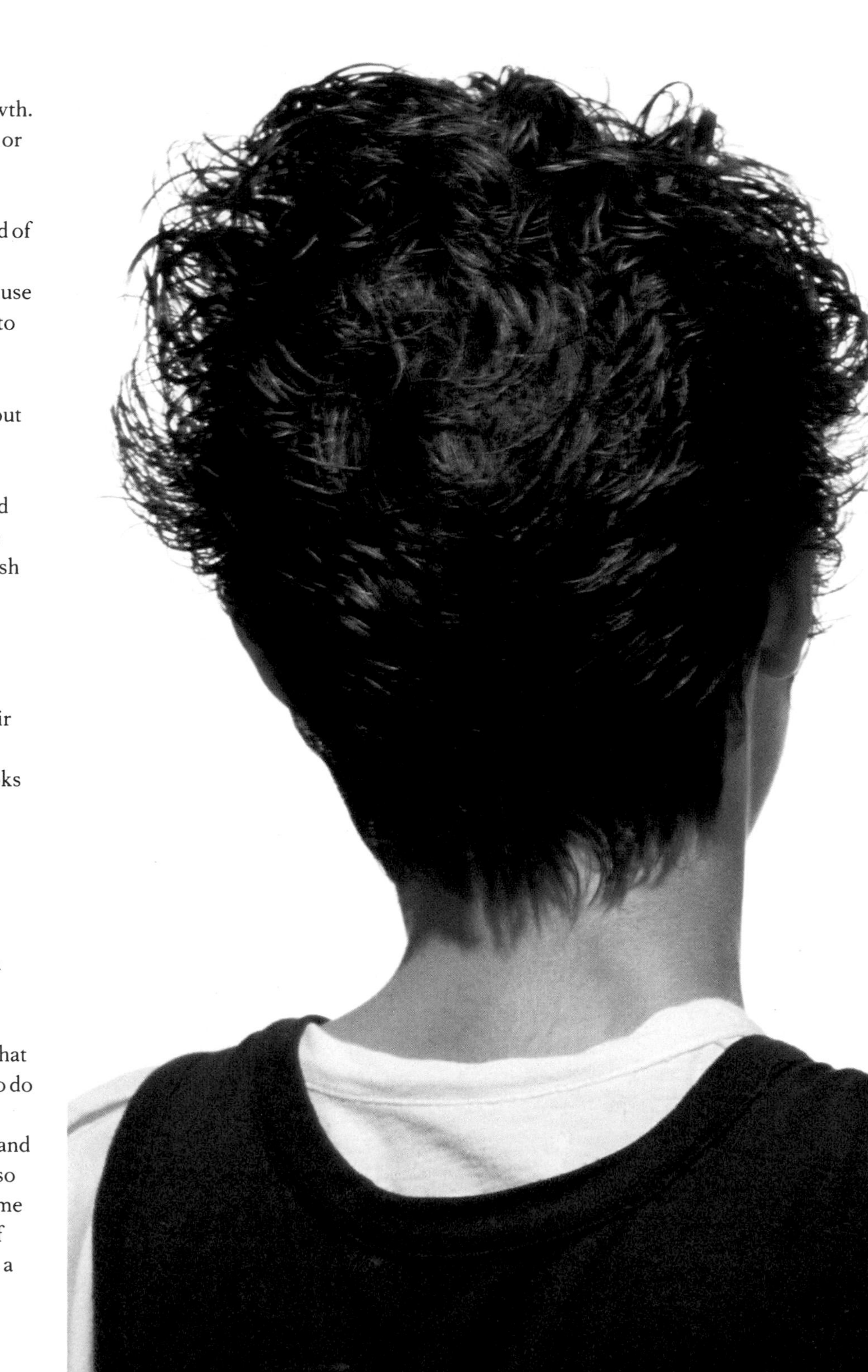

The cut of your hair is terribly important. Even long hair needs a good cut if it is going to look at its best. Ideally your hair should be cut according to the way that it grows, so that it is easy to look after when you have to do it yourself. If the style is complicated, watch the stylist carefully as he works and ask him to tell you how to look after it so that you can reproduce the effect at home and keep it looking good all the time. If you are the kind of person who prefers a wash-and-wear style to anything that needs a lot of attention, tell your hairdresser, who will take it into consideration.

If your hair is very fine, having a perm as well as a good cut will give it the body and 'lift' it lacks naturally.

Think about having your hair cut

about once every six weeks. After this, the style becomes unbalanced as the hair grows. Go regularly for a trim even if you are growing your hair. It is important that it should continue to look good while you are in the process of achieving the length that you want. Otherwise you may get impatient with the 'in between' stage and give up on your attempt to grow it.

Hair should not be over-brushed or combed, just enough to take the tangles out and put it into style. Brushes should be rubber-cushioned, with well-spaced, smooth plastic or real hair bristles. Both brushes and combs should be kept very clean – you can wash them at the same time as you wash your hair, using the same shampoo if you wish.

You can wash your hair as much as it seems to need – every day if your hair is very greasy and you use a mild shampoo. Choose a shampoo suggested for your hair type. You will know by the feel if it is greasy, dry or particularly fine. Finish with the right conditioner for your hair type, to smooth down the outer cuticle of the hair and give it shine.

Avoid using too much heat on your hair when styling. Heated rollers or heated tongs damage the hair by drying it out. They should never be used on wet hair. Brushing or combing wet hair too vigorously will stretch it so much that it breaks or splits. If your hair is very tangled, work from the tips up towards the roots getting out every tangle before proceeding higher. Use a plastic (not steel) comb with wide-set, round-ended teeth.

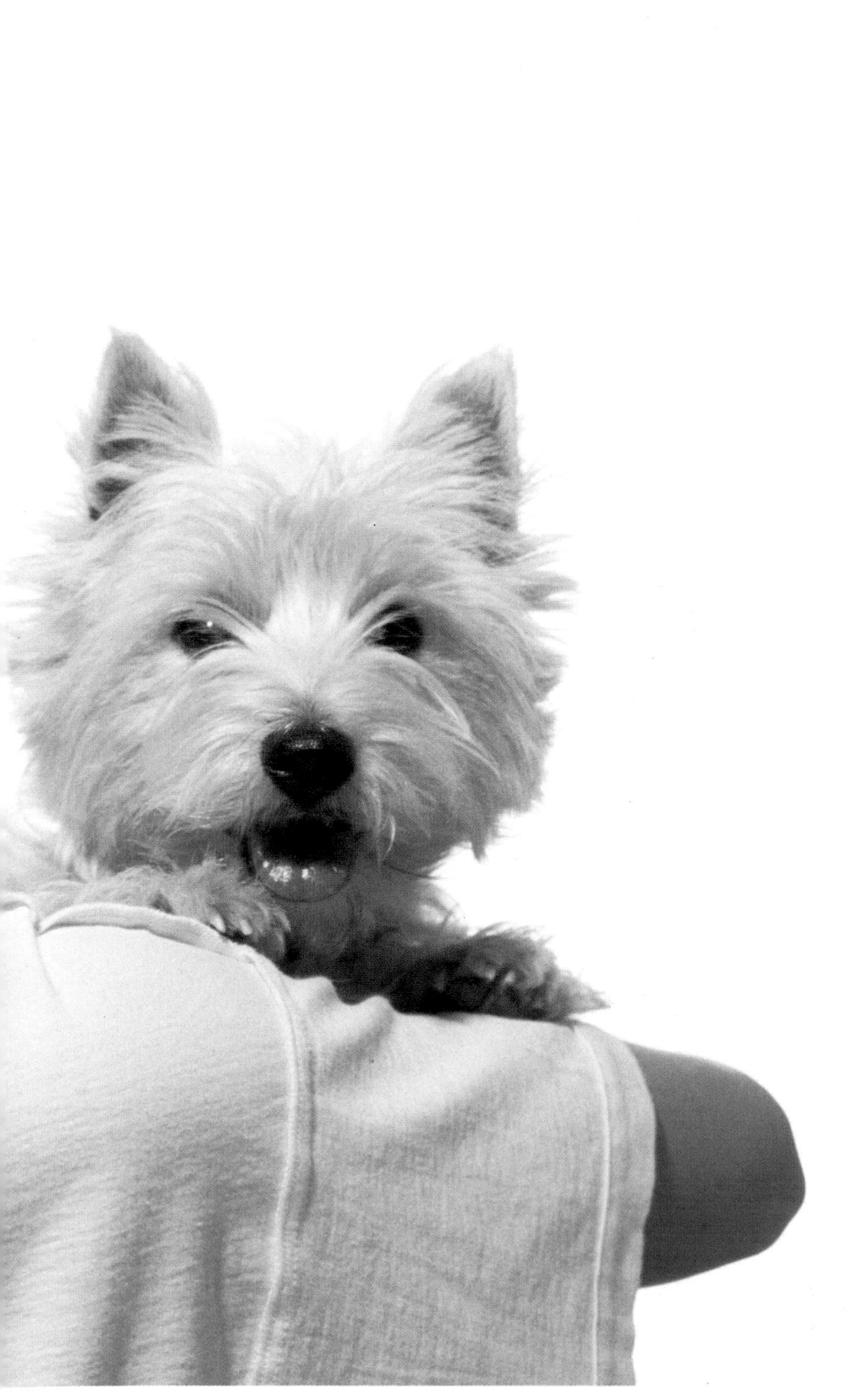

Dress: Comme des Garçons

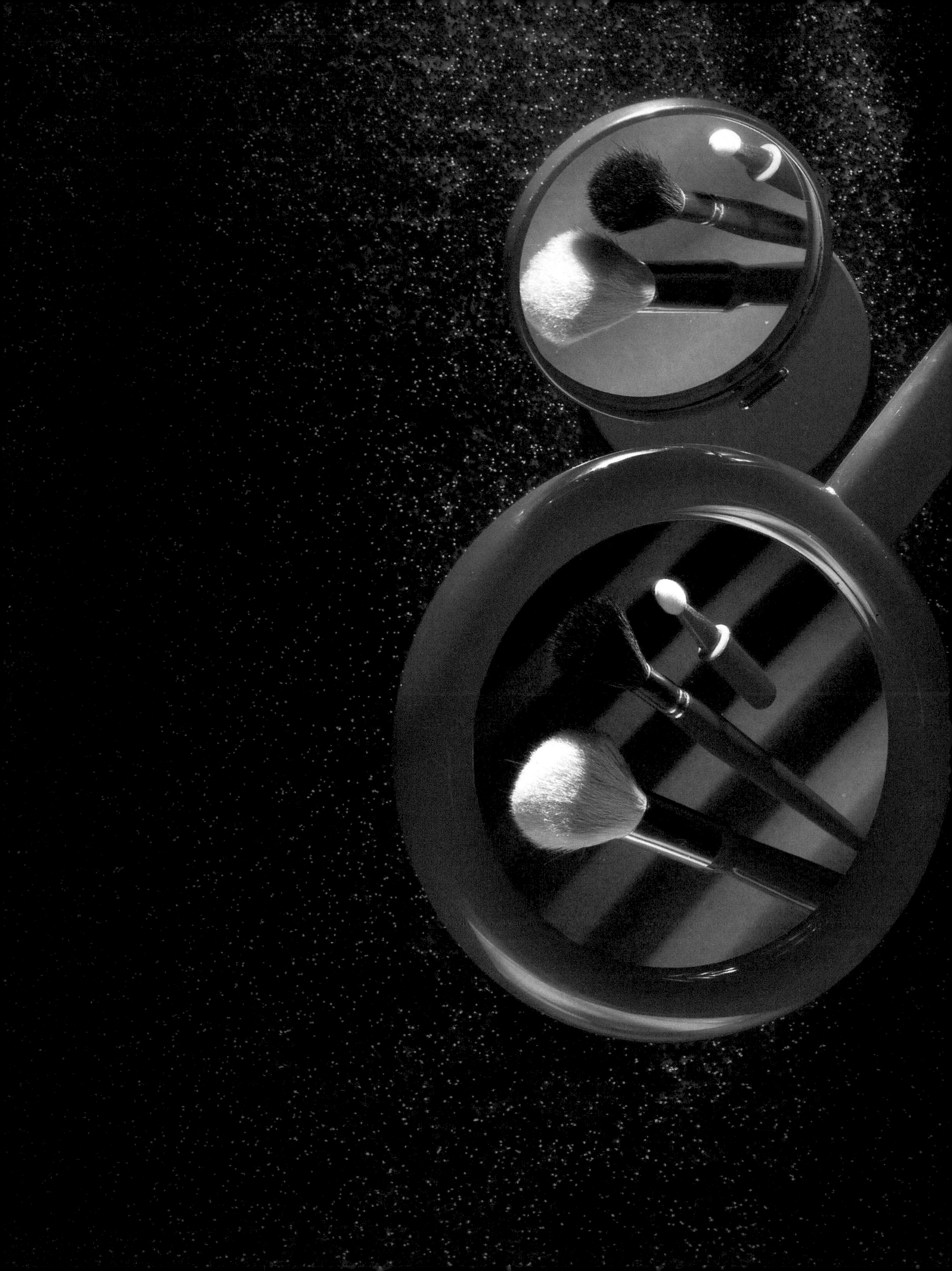

MAKING UP

Cosmetics are infinitely versatile — with the colours you choose you can go for a discreetly minimal look or something dramatic and bold. As a supplement to your wardrobe make-up is unbeatable: you can change your whole look by what you put on your face. Everyone can afford it — even the cheapest ranges have good colours and products — and it is good value: an expensive lipstick can last a year, which means it costs mere pennies a week. When you look good you feel good. Doctors now 'prescribe' make-up lessons for women who are depressed, because they know it is one of the nicest ways to boost morale. Try experimenting with new colours and ideas, or you will date yourself by sticking to a 'face' you have always applied. Above all, make-up should be fun.

FOUNDATION

A lightly tinted foundation evens up your skin tone, and appears to improve the texture of your skin, giving the illusion of a perfect complexion. It also provides the ideal base for blusher, powder and so on. It has the further advantage of giving your skin an extra layer to act as a barrier against dirt and dust. The choice of colours is wide, but to look natural choose the shade nearest your own skin tone rather than the colour you would like to be. Consistency varies, too, from very thin tinted liquids to solid blocks of colour. If in doubt, go for a lightweight liquid in a bottle or tube, which is suitable for every type of skin. As a general rule, oil-based foundations, which smooth on easily once in contact with warm skin, can be applied with your fingers. Water-based foundations can be put on with a cosmetic sponge.

There are other points to be considered when looking for a foundation for your special needs:

- Water-based foundation is a good choice for especially oily skin.
- Moisturized foundation, which is usually oil-based, will help dry skin.
- Hypo-allergenic foundations leave out ingredients, such as perfume, which may irritate sensitive skin.
- Medicated foundation may help young spotty skins, but can cause an allergic reaction on sensitive skin.
- Green-tinted foundation, used sparingly, can correct high colour.
- Gels and skin-tint liquids add colour and gloss to good, clear skin, but cannot correct uneven colour as effectively as a thicker foundation can.

CONCEALERS

These are skin-toned cover-ups that are thicker than foundation, and are used on certain areas of your face to cover dark shadows and blemishes. They come in a stick or tube in a limited range of colours — as few as two or three. Apply them with a brush, your finger, or straight from the stick. They can be used under or over foundation, or on their own. Special medicated concealers dry up spots as they hide them.

FACE POWDER

Powder fixes foundation by absorbing some of the surface oil. It makes the pores of the skin less apparent and gives it a finer and smoother finish. It comes in two forms, compressed or loose. Compressed powder, in a compact, is easier to carry around. Loose powder is a good way to achieve a perfect make-up at the beginning of the day. Touch up later with a compact or keep some loose powder in a small container in your handbag.

The main types of powder are transparent (which, because it is very light in colour, will not add colour to your face), and translucent (which means it is light-reflecting). Because most modern powders are finely ground they are translucent. Whether you use compressed or loose powder, choose one without much colour.

BLUSHERS

Blushers add colour to your skin and make your face glow. Blushers in cream, liquid, pencil and crayon form should be used on top of foundation or moisturizer, *not* over face powder. Powder blushers are meant to be used *after* face powder.

SHADERS & HIGHLIGHTERS

By using the principle of light and shade, shaders and highlighters subtly appear to alter the contours of the face. Darker colours with a matt finish deepen a hollow or make a feature recede; light and shiny colours highlight an area and make it stand out.

Contouring powders should be applied with a large soft brush; other types can be smoothed on with your fingers before putting on face powder.

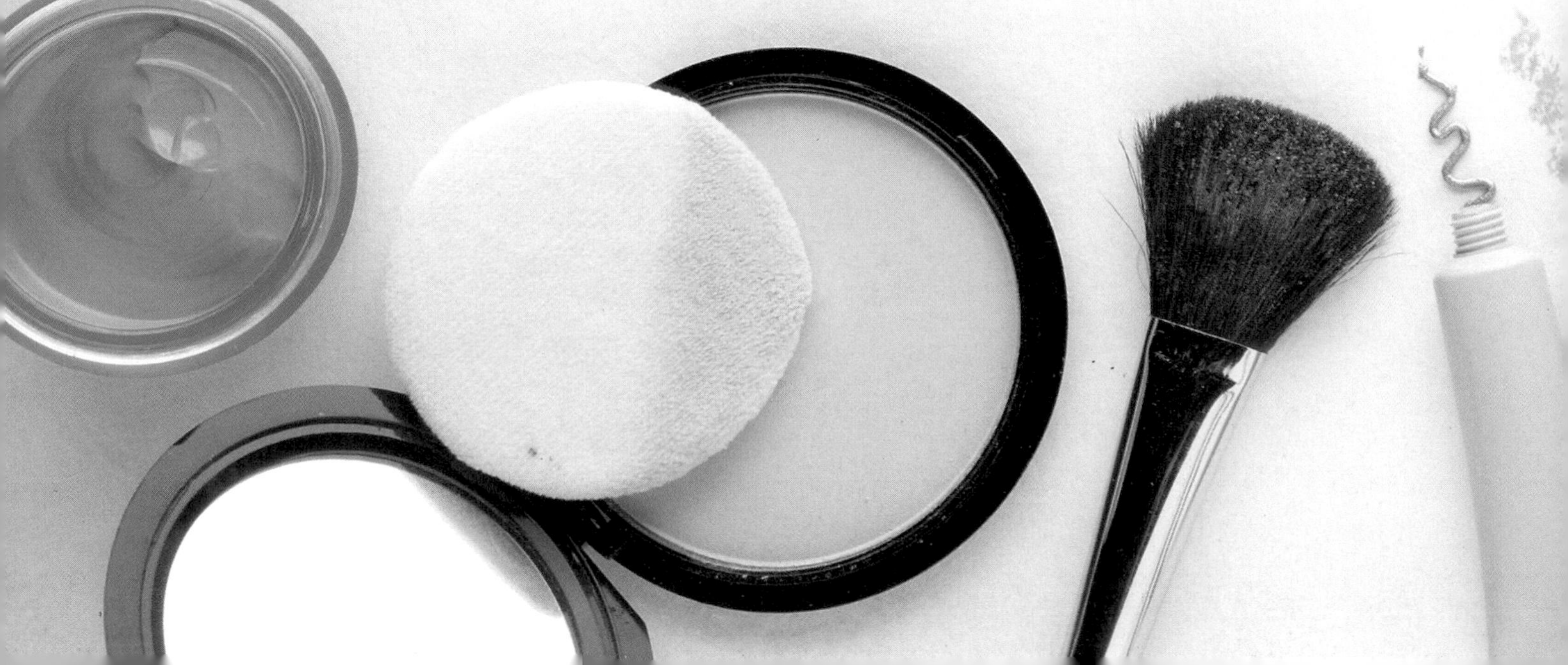

EYE MAKE-UP

Broadly divided into shadows, liners and mascara, eye make-up defines the eye with colour and shading. Every possible colour is obtainable – the depth and degree set the mood for your entire face.

Shadows come in the form of creams, sticks, liquids, gels, powders, watercolours, crayons or pencils. Choose whichever you find easiest to put on, but do not use crayon over a powdered area. If a pencil drags the delicate skin around your eyes, a base of foundation is needed to help it glide on easily.

Liners come as liquids, pencils, cakes or wands, and should usually be applied thinly with a brush to emphasize the natural line of your eye.

Mascara is most commonly found in wand form, but you can also buy cake mascara which is mixed with a little water and put on with a brush. All mascara adds colour and thickness to your lashes. Mascaras are formulated with certain properties: some are waterproof, some have fine filaments to add length to your lashes, others can help hold moisturizer on the lashes.

LIP COLOUR

Lipsticks, lip glosses and crayons not only add colour to your mouth, but keep the sensitive skin of your lips moist and shielded from the elements.

Pencils offer the most concentrated colour, and are used to outline the mouth. Lipsticks are solid colour dispersed in a wax base. Creamy and moisturizing, they are not especially long-lasting. For lipstick to stay on all day it would have to be made to the old-fashioned formula which was quite drying. Lip-colour fixatives are now available which hold the colour well. Gels and glosses have a high grease content, adding lots of shine with the colour. Lipsticks are often used straight from the stick, but a brush gives a clearer outline and longer-lasting finish.

EQUIPMENT

Trying to apply expensive, carefully chosen products with your fingers, cotton wool and a couple of cotton buds is wasteful. The essentials are:

Light – always put on your make-up in the best and strongest light available. If it is daytime make-up sit by a window; for night-time and party make-up use good, white artificial light. Never 'fool' yourself by making up in dim or pink and flattering light.

Magnifying mirror – you need a clear close-up view of what you're doing if it is to look professional and neatly finished.

Brushes – collect different-sized brushes for each kind of make-up: a fat one for loose powder; a smaller, but bushy brush for applying blusher and contour powder and a clutch of small brushes for eye make-up application and blending in; last but not least, a lip brush.

Eyebrow and eyelash combs – eyelash combs separate your lashes. Eyebrow brushes smooth down your brows; so will an old toothbrush.

Sponges – for applying foundation you will need either a natural sponge or a baby sponge cut into small pieces.

Powder puffs – velour is very soft and, because you can wash it, hygienic.

Pencil sharpener – a sharp point on your lip and eye pencils is essential. Buy a sharpener of the right size.

CARE OF EQUIPMENT

Keep all equipment scrupulously clean. Wash anything washable regularly. Brushes made from real hair pose a problem, as washing makes the hairs splay out and ruins them. Dry-cleaning fluid, used according to instructions, is the best way to clean them. Keep all your brushes bristle upwards in a pot, even those that come in a container with a specific product, or the bristles will become squashed.

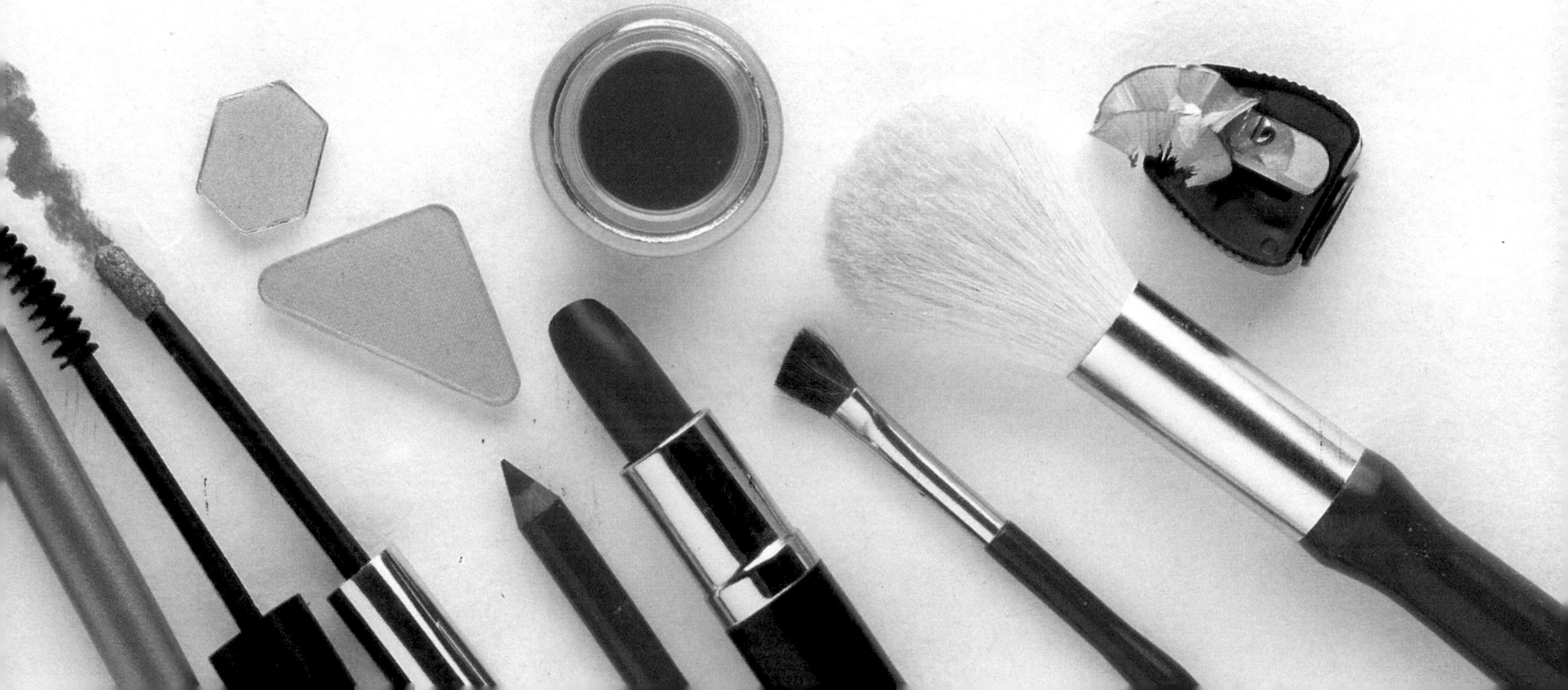

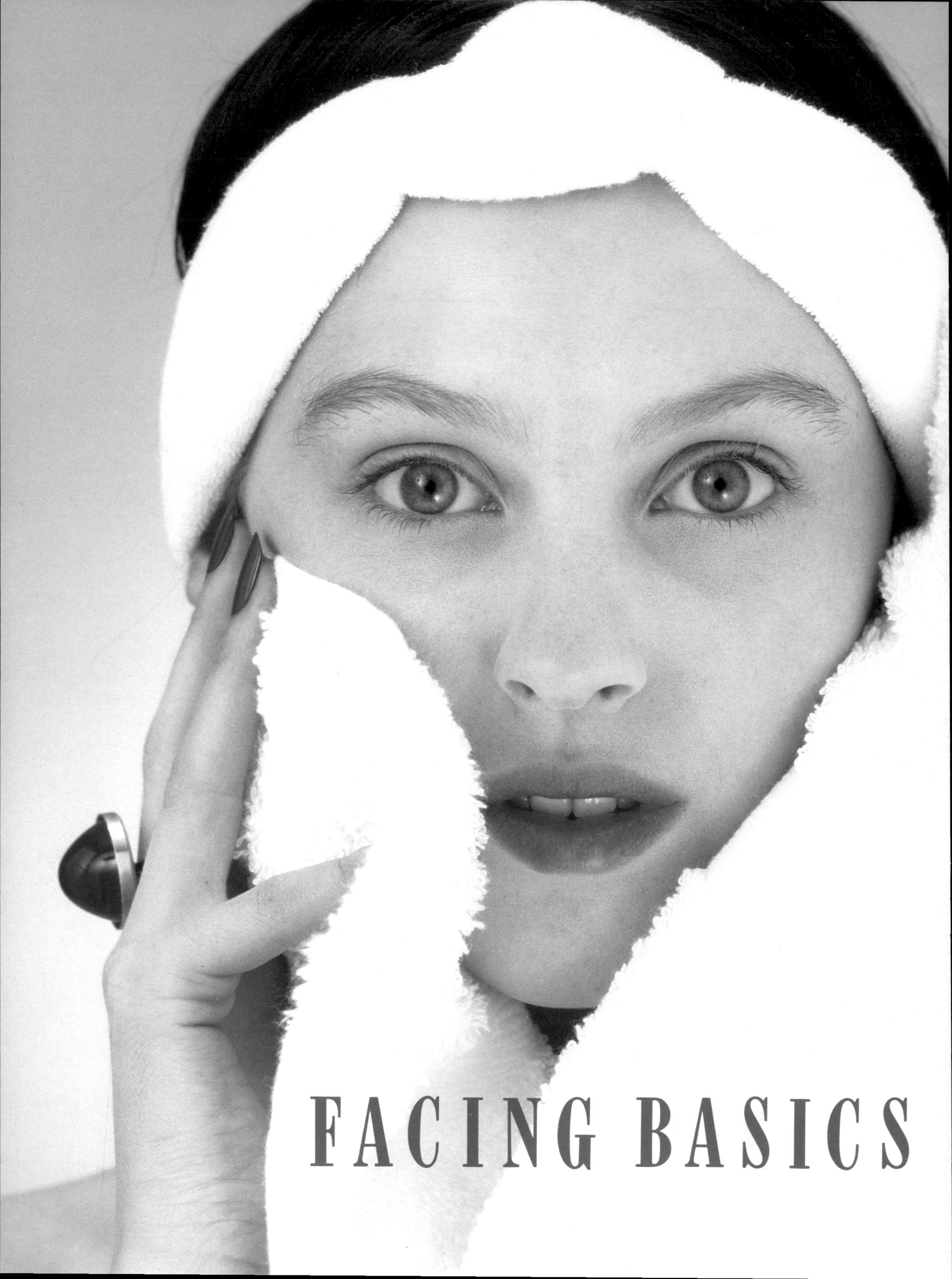

FACING BASICS

This is a step by step guide to making up your face to achieve a look that is sophisticated but subtle and using a simple collection of cosmetics. Although it is understated, the effect is striking: never underestimate the importance of applying each item of make-up with great care and patience, working in good light and with a magnifying mirror so that you can check as you go that the finish is neat and smooth.

You can see on these pages how each stage of this make-up was achieved, and what is the best and most professional way to apply the various products used. Careful blending in at every stage is essential. This 'face' suits most colourings, but you can adapt it when applying your own make-up — choosing the colours you like or the ones that suit you best while duplicating the techniques demonstrated by our model Susie.

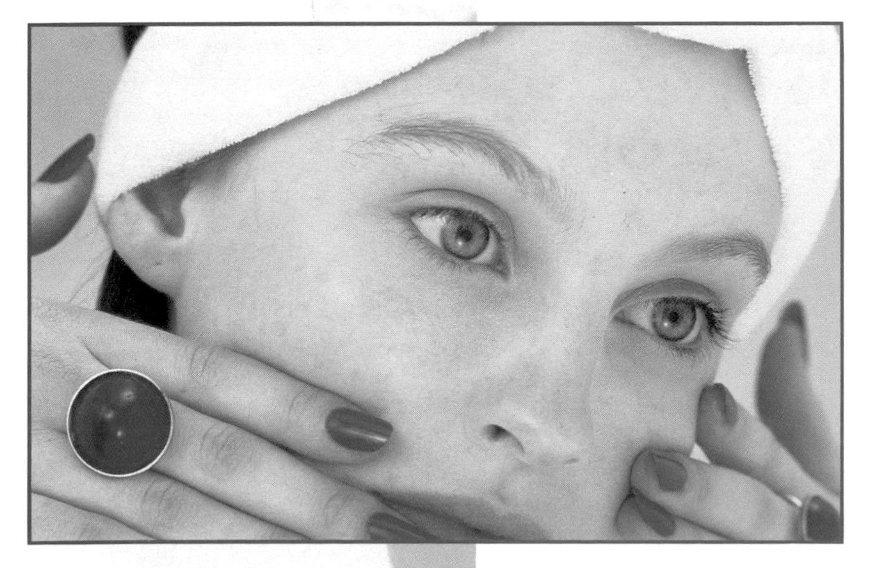

Susie prepares to make up with a face that is superclean, gently patted dry on a soft towel.

1 Take a good look at your face before you begin, to assess aspects that may need special attention.

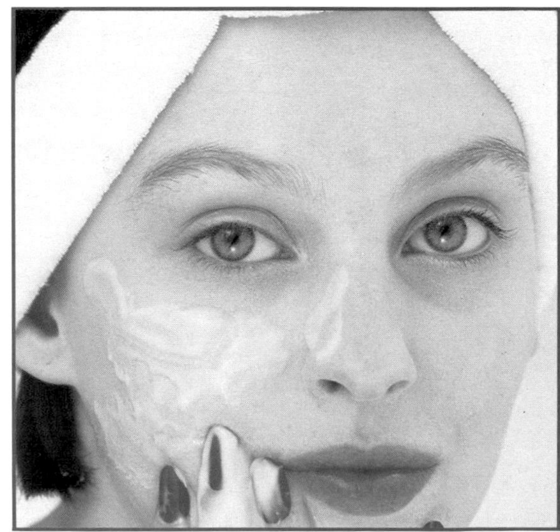

2 **Moisturizer** Apply suitable moisturizer liberally all over your face and throat. Blend it in well until it has disappeared into your skin.

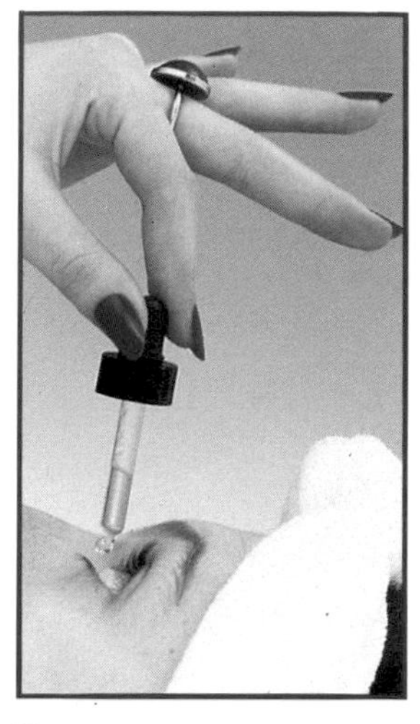

3 **Eyedrops** If your eyes are feeling sore or tired, use a drop of eye-refreshing liquid to revive them

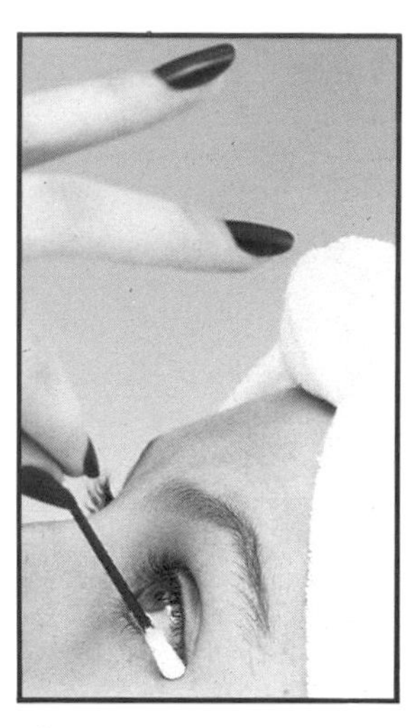

4 Use a cottonbud to absorb any excess liquid from the corner of your eyes

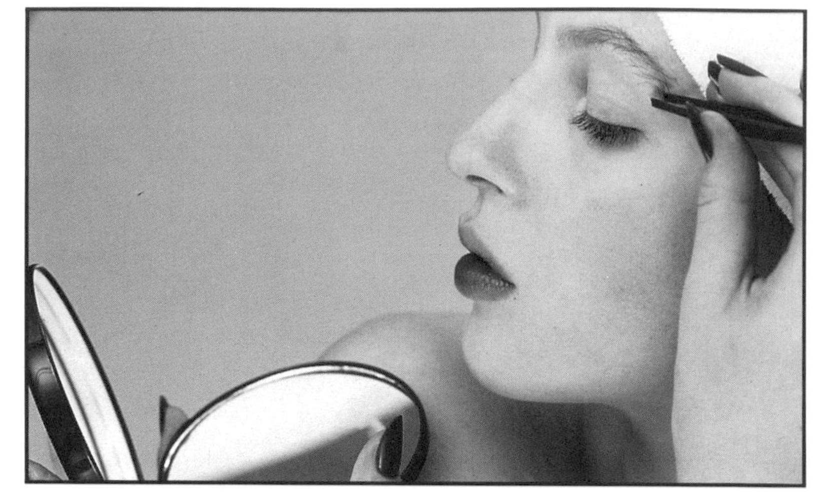

5 **Tweezers** If you have the odd stray eyebrow hair, pull it out before you start to apply any make-up. Powder and powder eye-shadow will make stray hairs more noticeable, and if you leave tweezing until your make-up is complete it may make your eyes water and spoil what you've done

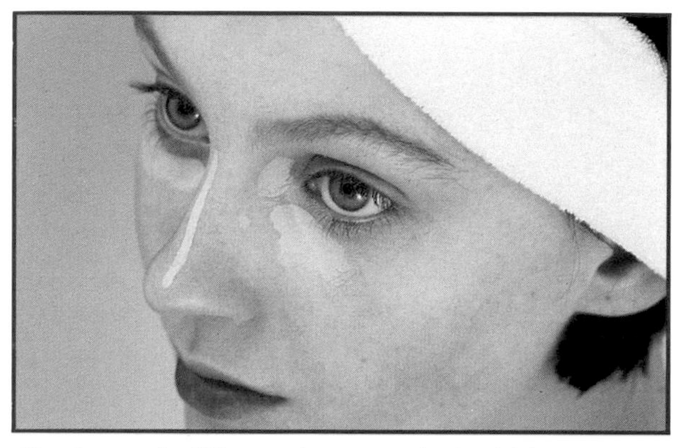

9 **Concealer** We are using a concealer in stick form to cover blemishes on the face and dark shadows under the eyes. Stroke it on the areas where you have to use it, either straight from the stick or with a brush

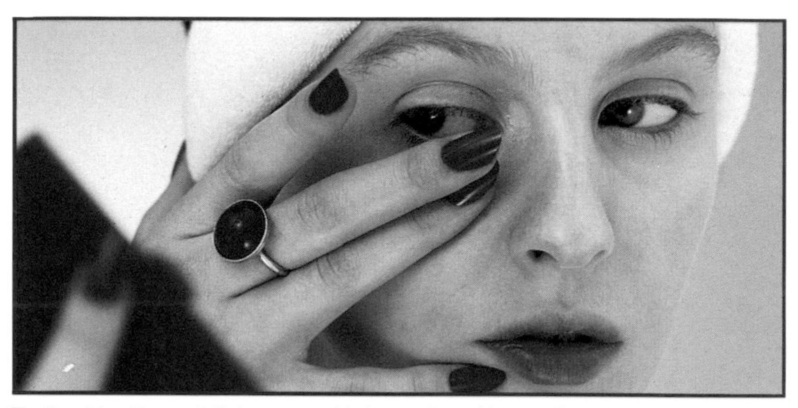

10 Blend it carefully into your skin by patting with your fingertip. Use the third finger of your hand if possible because you can exert the least pressure. Don't rub the cream in — this will be damaging to the delicate skin around the eye — just press or pat it

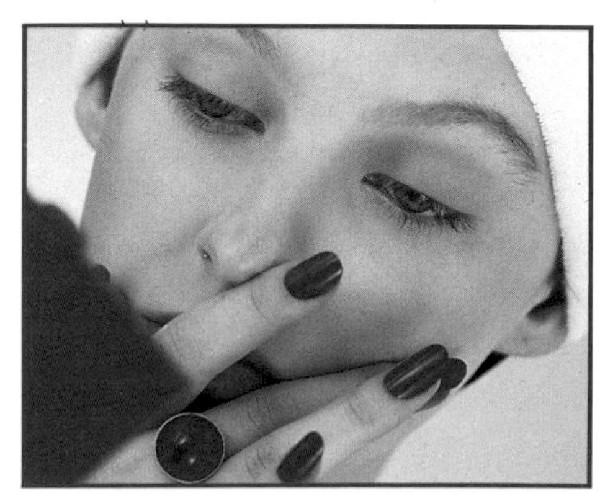

13 Blend the blusher over your cheek to give your face a soft glow. Blend with fingertips so that there are no hard lines. Wipe your fingers on a tissue

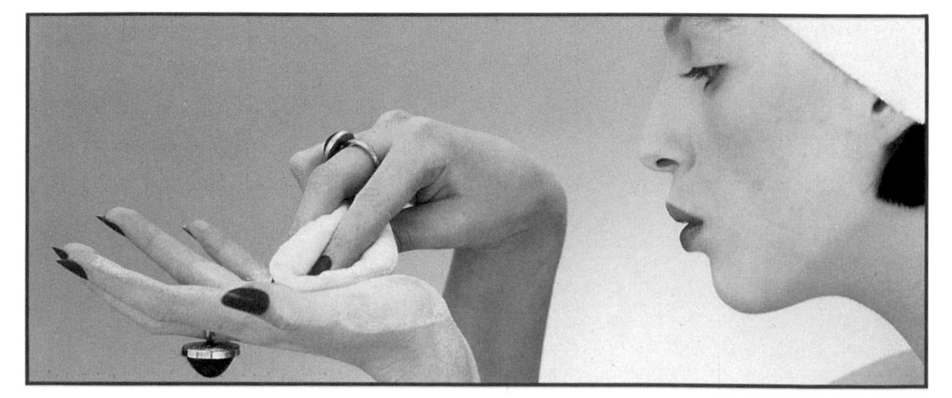

14 **Powder** Now's the time to set the foundation with face powder. Use a 'transparent' powder, that is, one which is very fine and light in colour. Using a powder puff, pat the loose powder into the palm of your hand. For perfect coverage you will need slightly more than you think; the excess will be brushed away

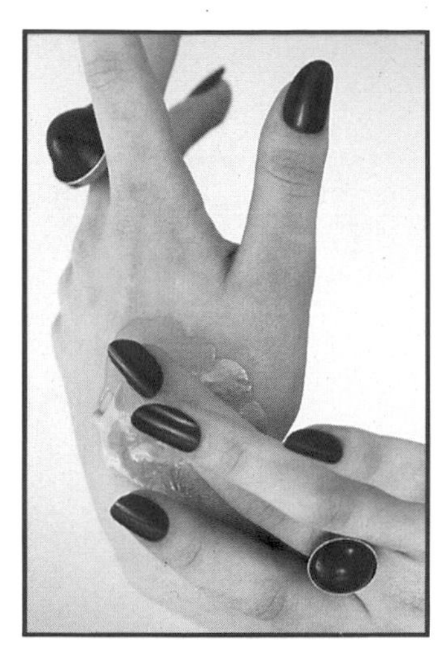

6 **Foundation** If you are mixing colours to match your skin tone, blend them on the back of your hand

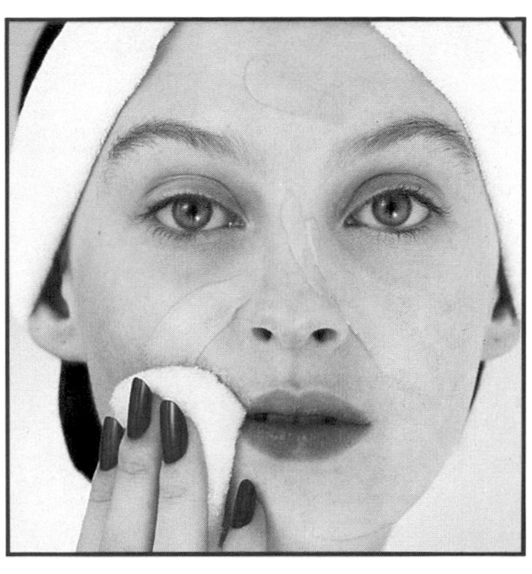

7 Smooth the foundation over your face and throat with a slightly damp cosmetic sponge. Do not drag it over your face, but apply gentle pressure in short sweeps

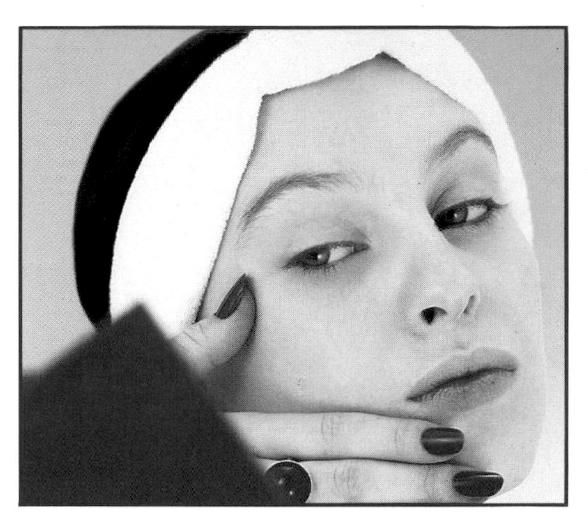

8 Work in a good light, blending in the foundation with your fingertips. Check that none is stuck in your hairline, eyebrows or so on, that it continues under your chin and that you have not missed any bits

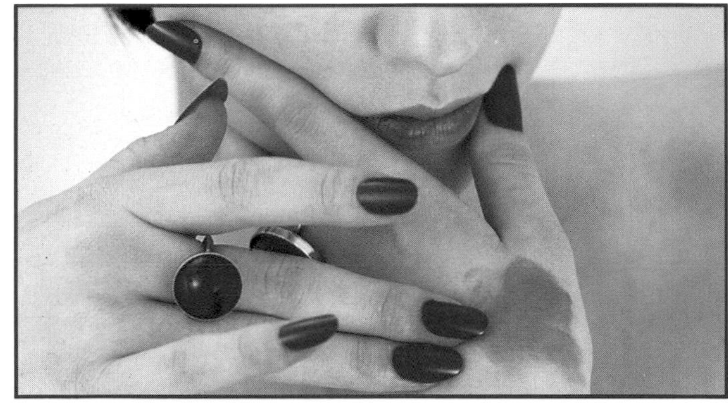

11 **Cream blusher** Cream blusher must be used before face powder. Soften a little of the blusher on the back of your hand to make it easier to use and to ensure that you do not put too much straight on your face

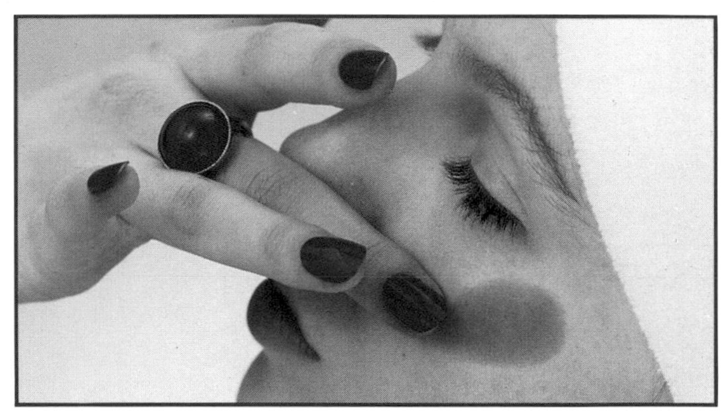

12 Smooth it on your cheeks in a teardrop shape, with the wider part at the outer edge, narrowing towards the centre of your face

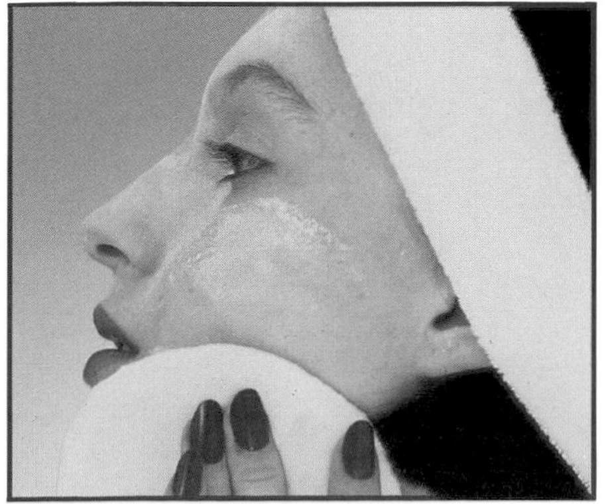

15 Press the powder all over your face with a clean puff. Never rub, or you'll streak the foundation. Too much around the eye may emphasize lines

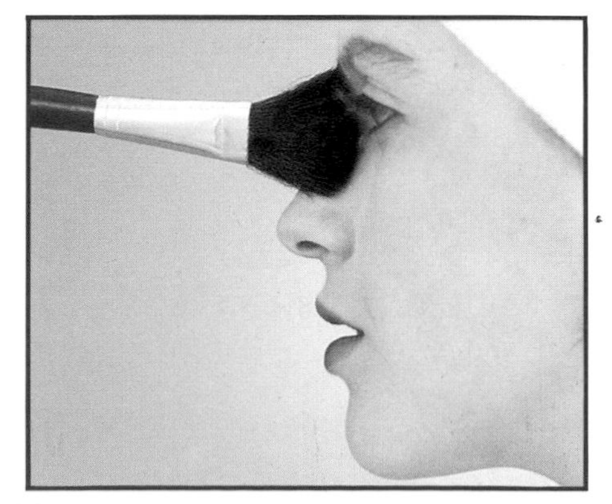

16 Brush off the surplus powder with the other side of the powder puff or a powder brush. Work downwards to avoid fluffing up tiny facial hairs

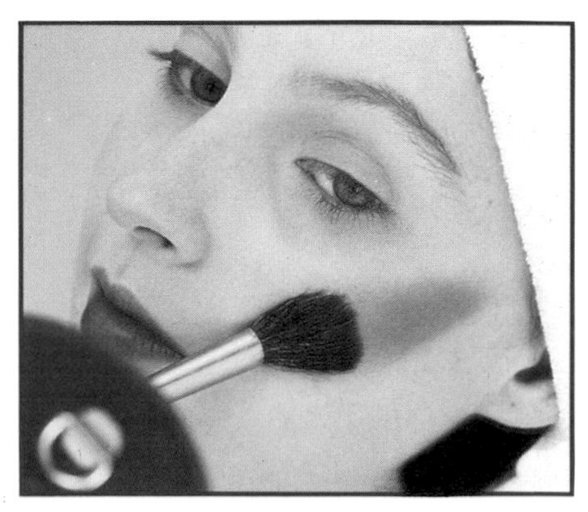

17 **Powder blusher** If you are using powder blusher, fluff on a little now. Apply in a teardrop shape, and blend with a thick brush or puff

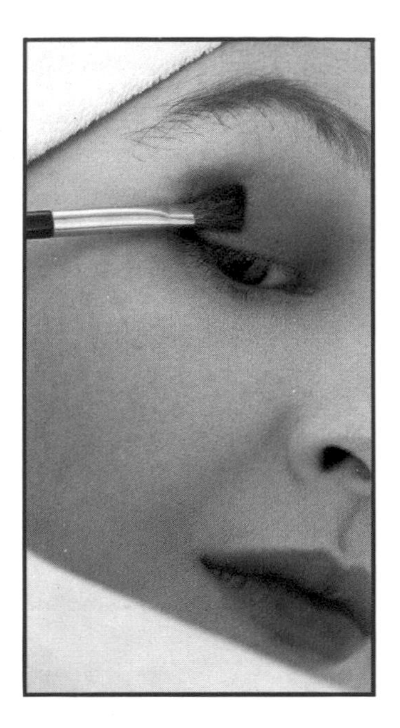

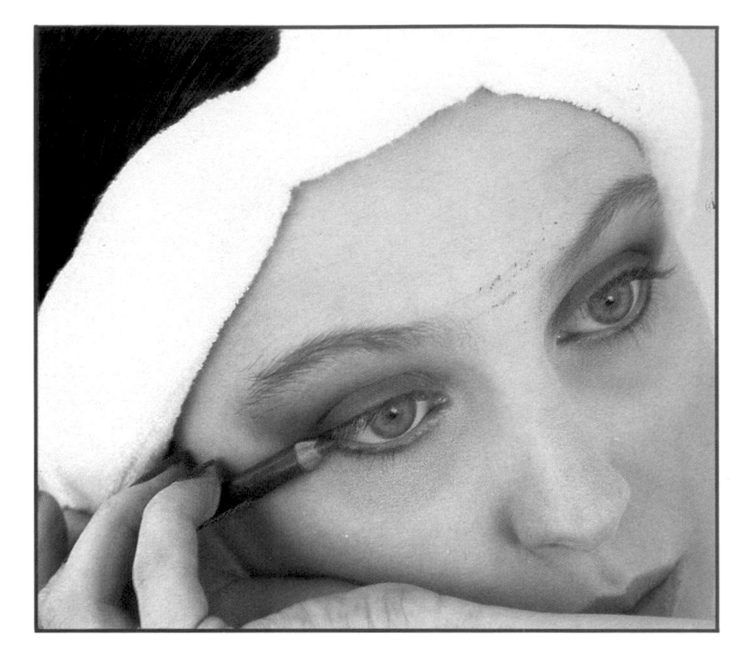

18 **Eyes** Blend taupe brown powder eyeshadow over the eyelids with a straight-edged brush

19 Using a darker tone on the outer eyelid, make a curved triangle shape, working inwards

20 With a grey pencil, draw a line close to the lashes on the outer edge of the upper eyelid, flaring slightly upwards and outwards. Repeat on the lower lid, and soften the pencil line with fingertip and a soft straight-edged brush

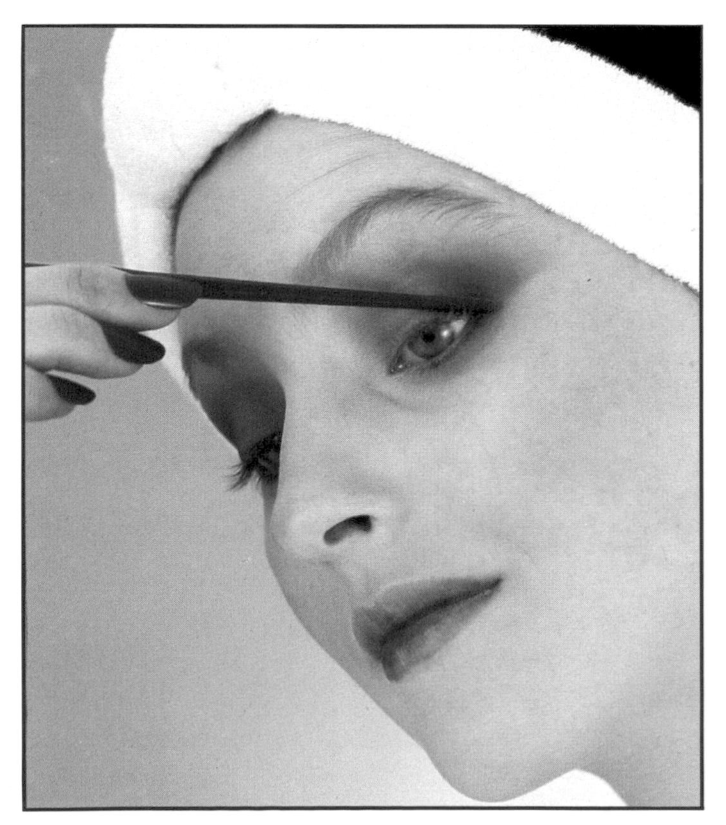

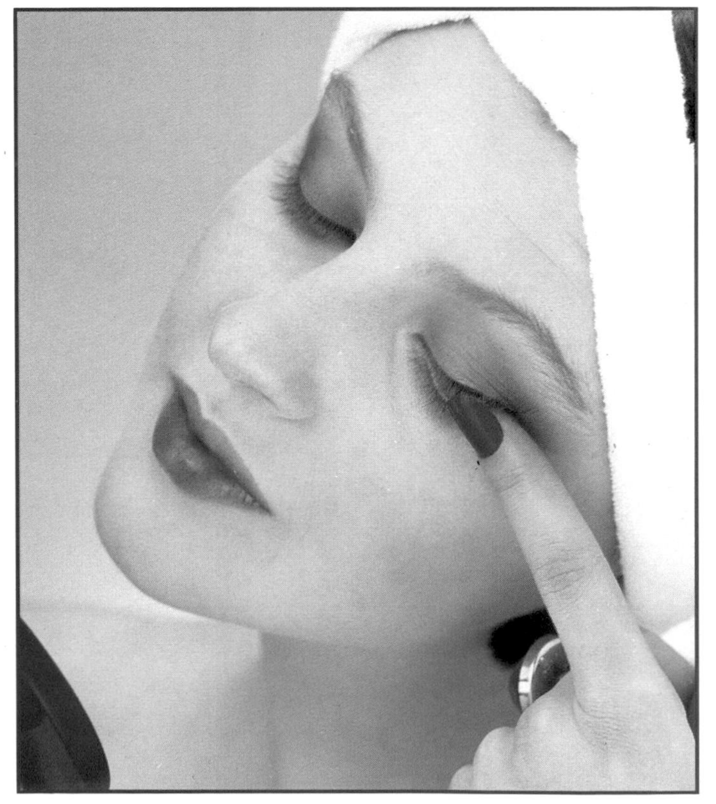

24 Use the brush-end as an applicator to place the false lashes at the outer corner of the eye. You need a steady hand — rest your elbow on a table if it helps. Some people prefer to put lashes on with tweezers

25 Put the lashes as close as you can to the natural line of your own eyelashes so that they merge together. When they are in place, push the lashes upwards with your fingernail. Let the glue dry for a moment before the next step

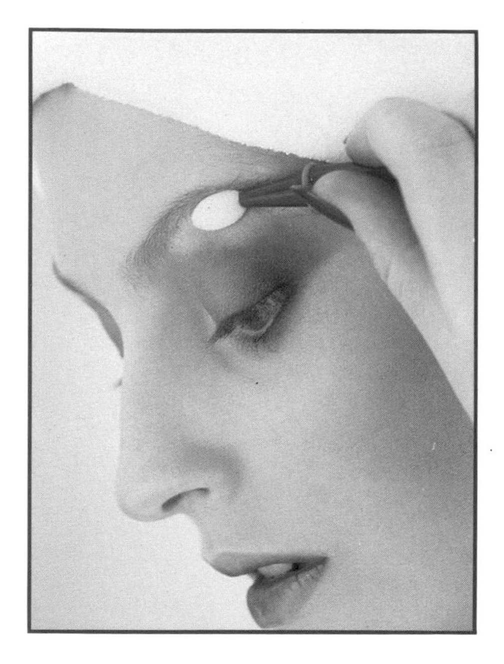

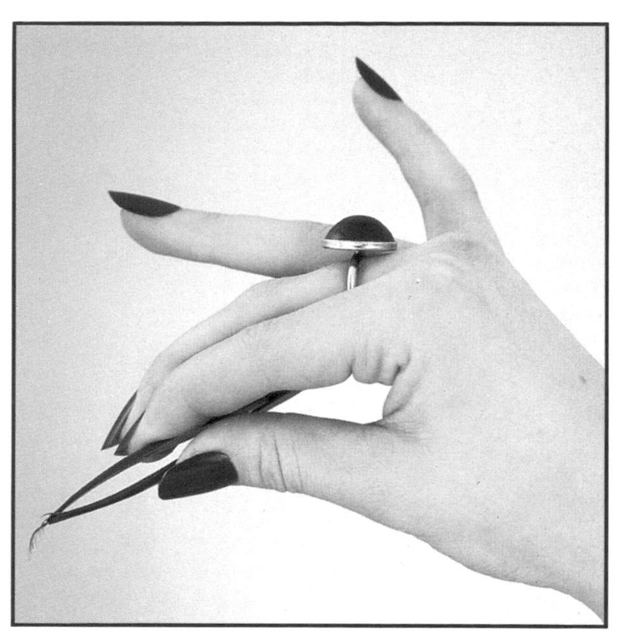

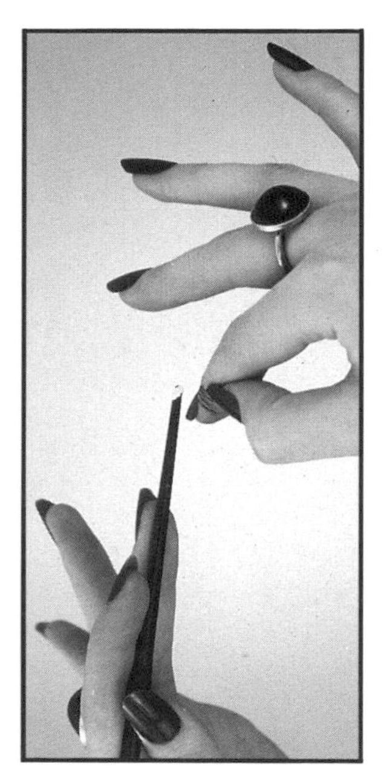

21 Apply powder highlighter under the browbone with a brush. Blend it in carefully with a sponge applicator. Check that your eyes 'match'

22 **The eye opener** Make your eyes wider by fixing a very few fake lashes to the outer corner of your eyes. Nip the end off a set of false lashes or use sections cut from a strip

23 Apply glue with the end of a brush to the lashes. When dry, the glue is transparent

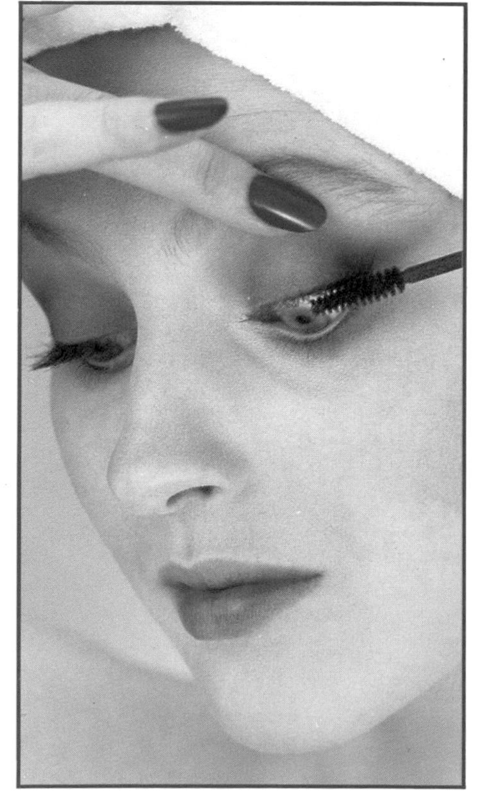

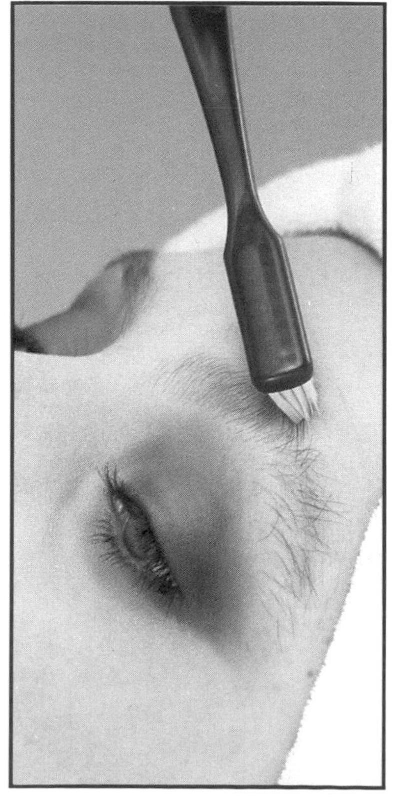

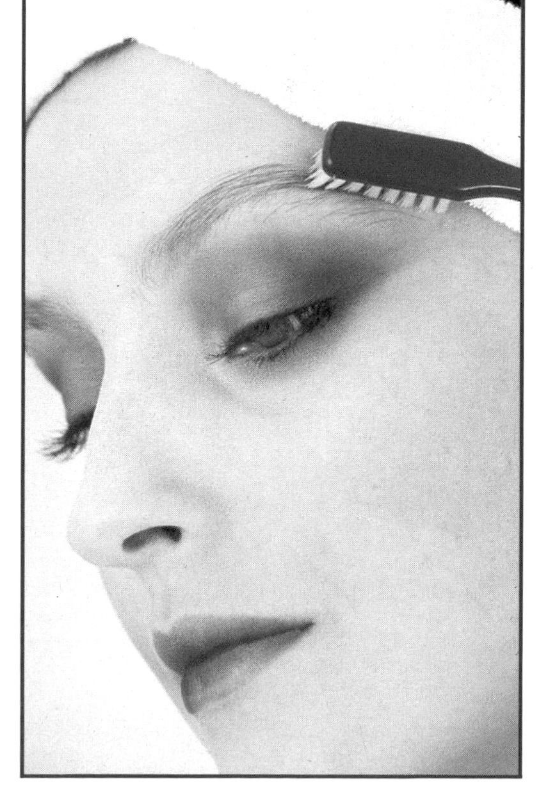

26 Apply mascara with a wand to the upper lashes first, looking slightly downwards. After putting mascara on the lower lashes, separate with a tiny comb

27 Using a medium toothbrush, brush the eyebrows against the direction of growth to remove any traces of make-up

28 Then brush in the right direction for a neat and finished line. You can get combined eyelash combs/eyebrow brushes which are quite useful additions to your make-up bag

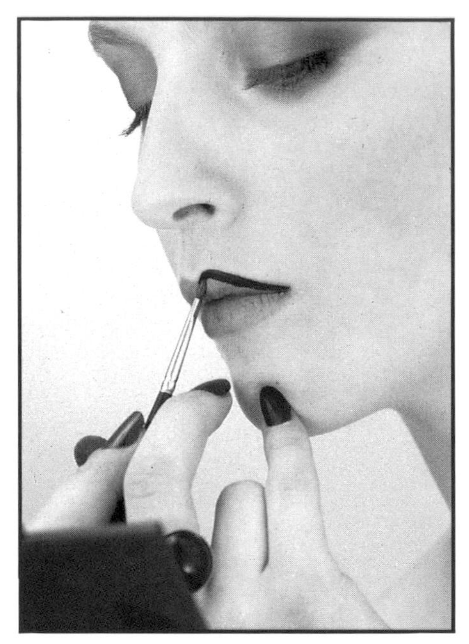

29 Lips Carefully draw the outline of your natural lip shape using a lip brush. Steady your hand on your chin. It takes practice, but this is a technique well worth learning

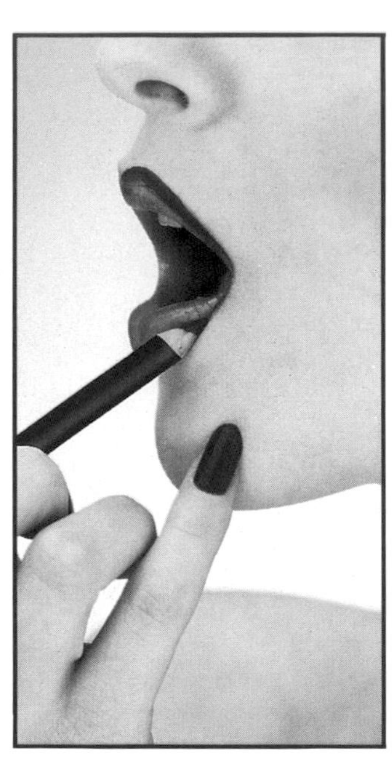

30 Some people find it easier to use a pencil sharpened to a fine point. Keep to the natural outline

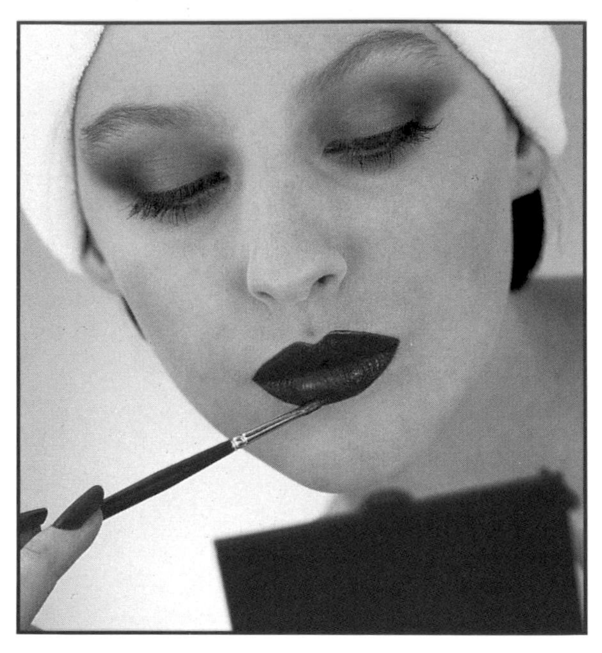

31 Fill in the outline with a brush, mixing colours (on the back of your hand) to get exactly the shade you want. We made clear scarlet even more vivid with a touch of orangey-red

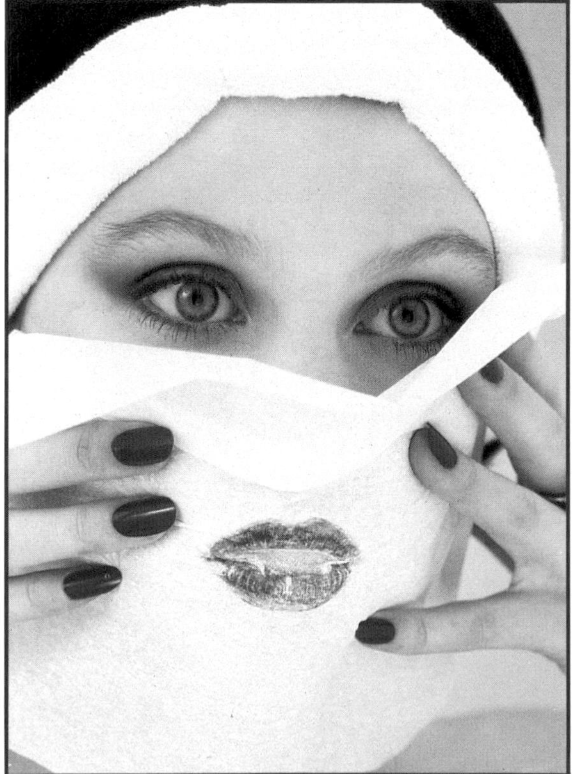

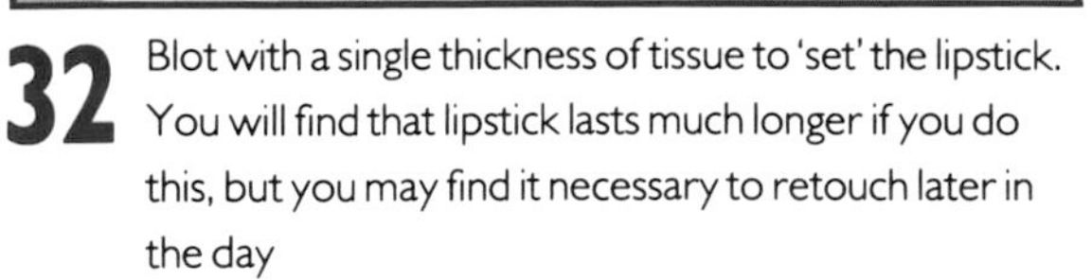

32 Blot with a single thickness of tissue to 'set' the lipstick. You will find that lipstick lasts much longer if you do this, but you may find it necessary to retouch later in the day

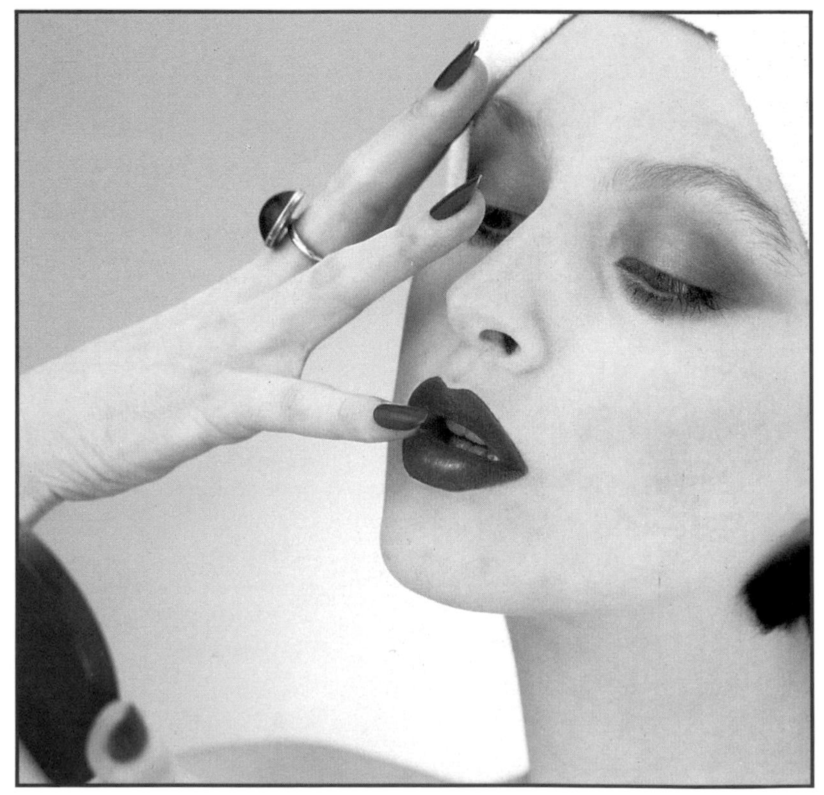

33 To add gleam and make your mouth look full and soft, stroke on a touch of soft pink lipstick to the centre of the lower lip. Opposite, the finished look – perfect face and immaculate hair

Dress: Betty Jackson · Jewellery: Garry Wright & Sheila Teague · Rings: Monty Don ·

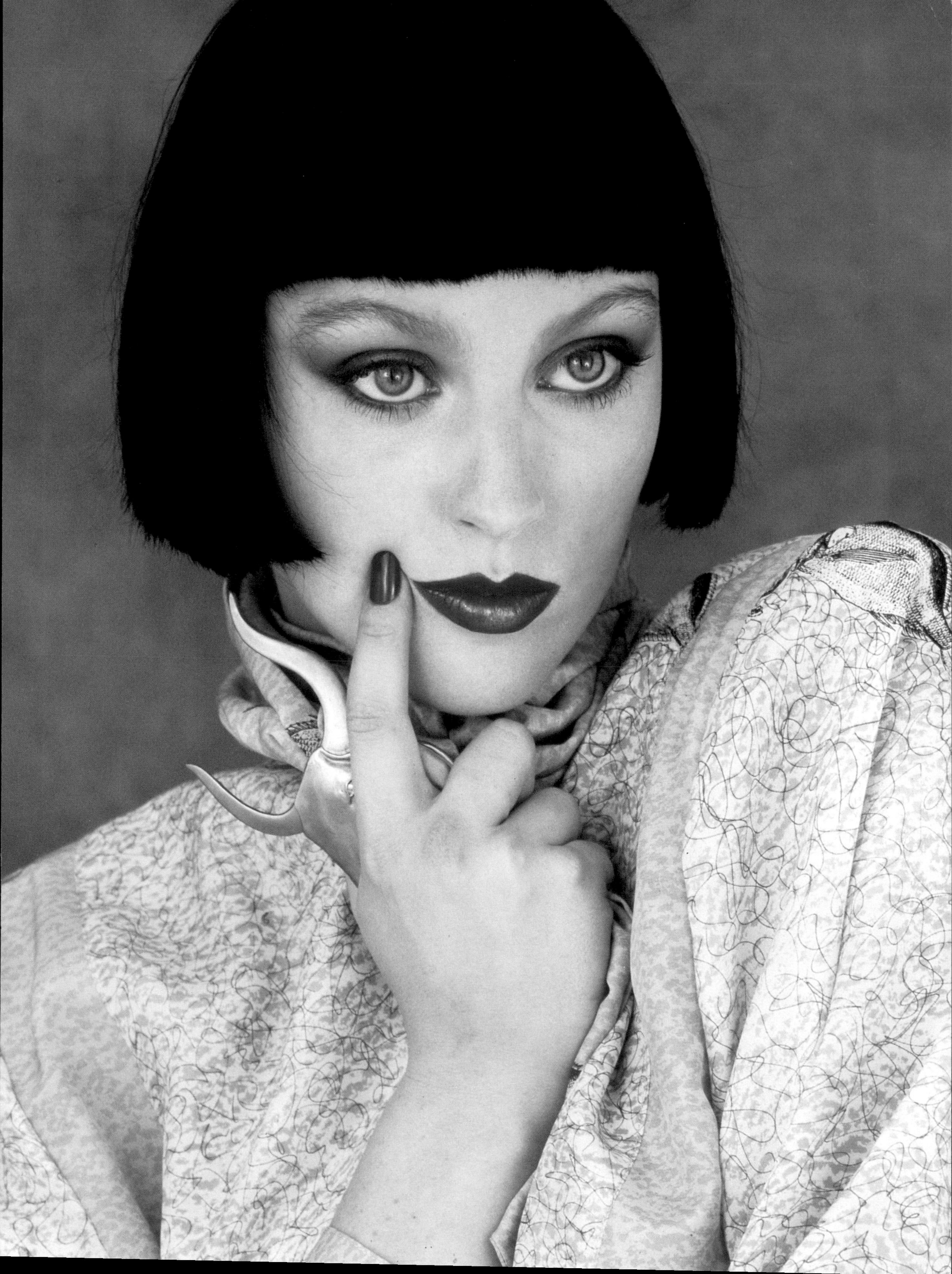

TIPS

Make-up is more than basic technique and a feel for colour. There are some tricks of the trade known almost exclusively to professional make-up artists and models. Here are some of my favourites. Remember to practise them thoroughly before you add them to your repertoire – don't try a 'trick' for the first time on a special occasion. And bear in mind that the greatest professional effect relies on no trick at all, but on patience. That's because the most successful make-up is blended with care and thoroughness so that there are no harsh lines, and colours naturally mix and flow together.

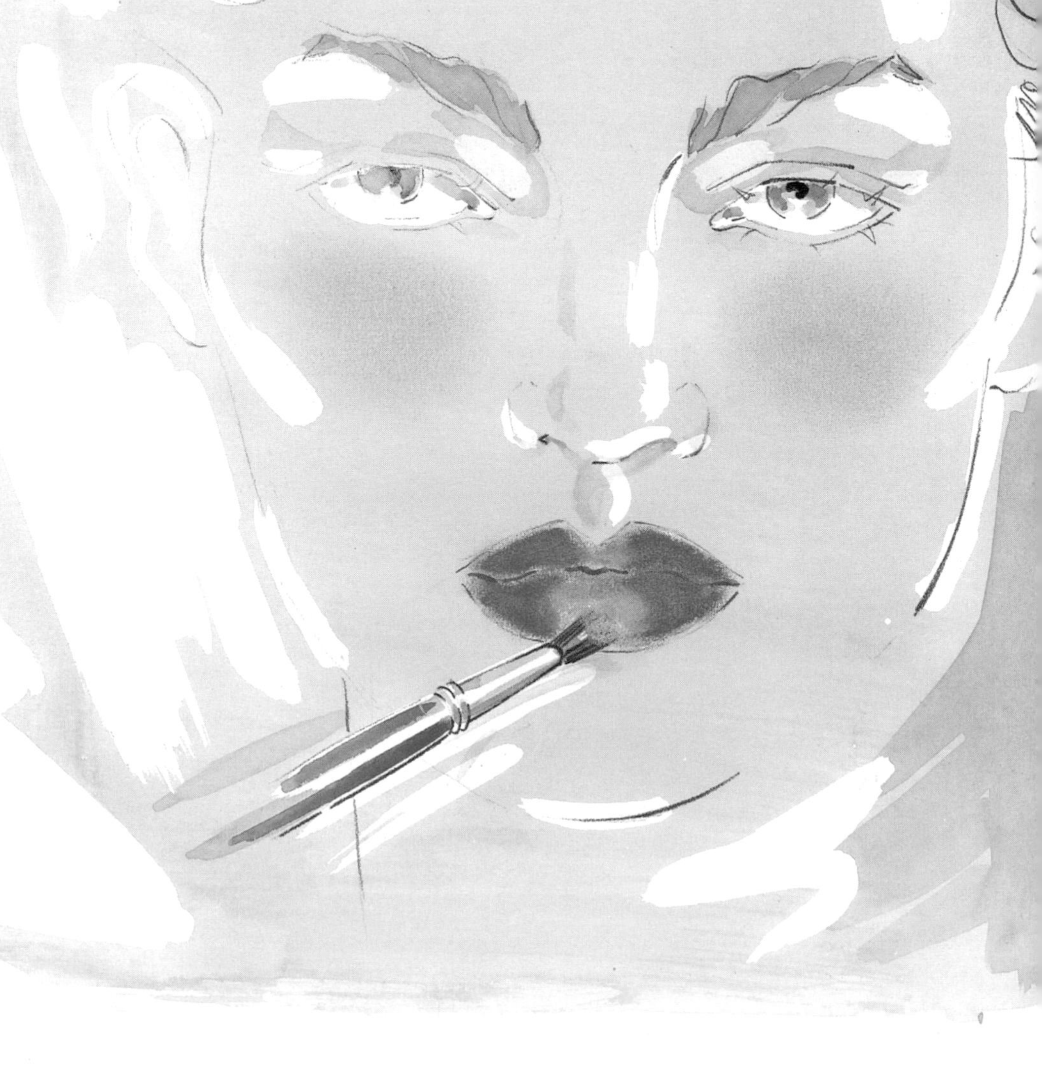

1 Make your mouth look fuller by highlighting your lips. Use a lighter shade of lipstick, or put a touch of foundation over the top of the colour on the centre of your upper and lower lips

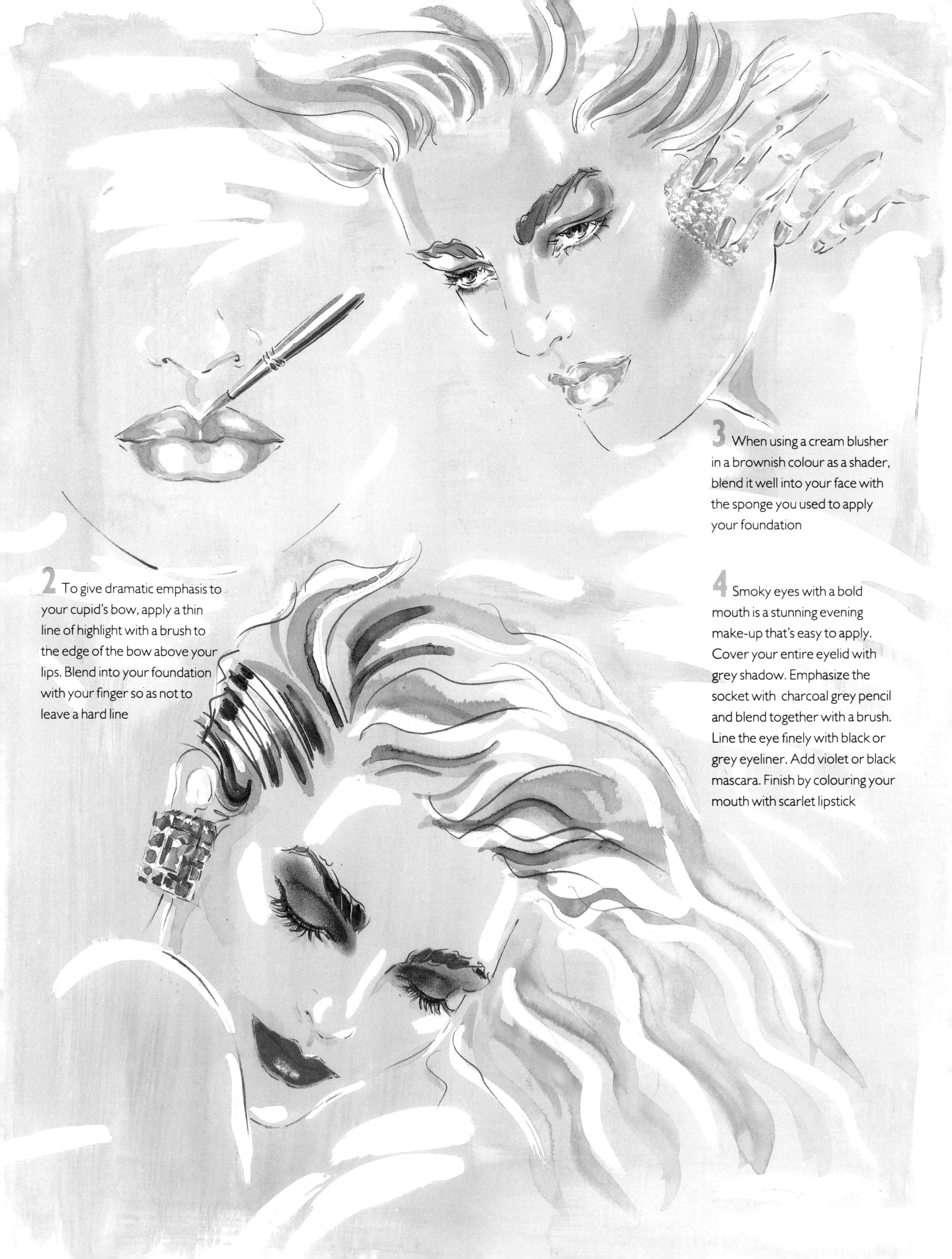

2 To give dramatic emphasis to your cupid's bow, apply a thin line of highlight with a brush to the edge of the bow above your lips. Blend into your foundation with your finger so as not to leave a hard line

3 When using a cream blusher in a brownish colour as a shader, blend it well into your face with the sponge you used to apply your foundation

4 Smoky eyes with a bold mouth is a stunning evening make-up that's easy to apply. Cover your entire eyelid with grey shadow. Emphasize the socket with charcoal grey pencil and blend together with a brush. Line the eye finely with black or grey eyeliner. Add violet or black mascara. Finish by colouring your mouth with scarlet lipstick

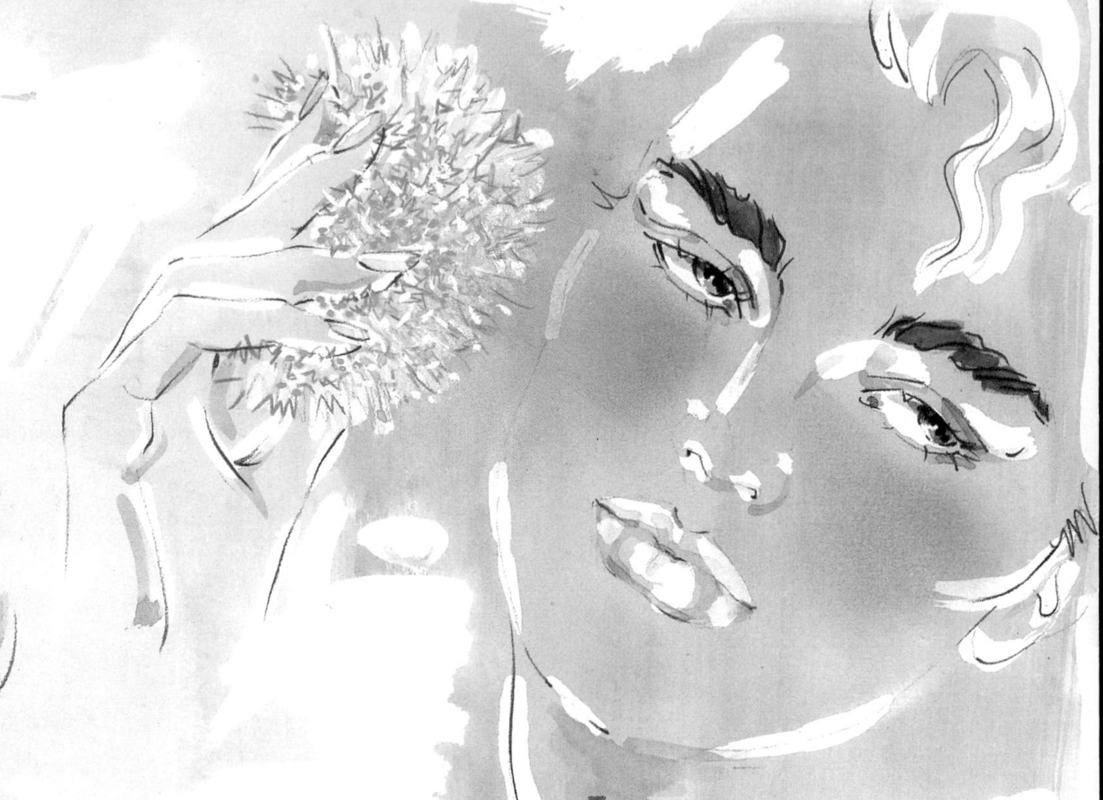

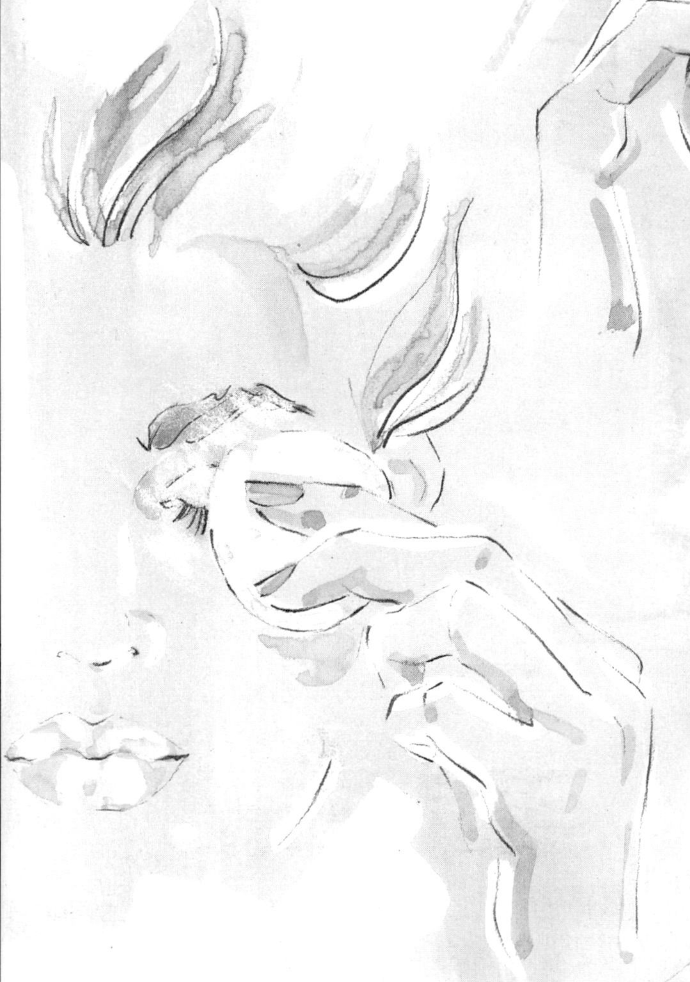

5 If you want to tone down very red cheeks, use a light dusting of green face powder Apply sparingly in very good light. (Red cheeks look better than green cheeks!)

6 To thicken eyelashes without using mascara with added filaments (which I hate!) powder your eyelashes with face powder before applying ordinary mascara. Do this after blending in your eyeshadow colours as the powder will also help set them. Apply the mascara to the topside of the upper lashes first, then the underside. When they are dry, comb out well with an eyelash comb

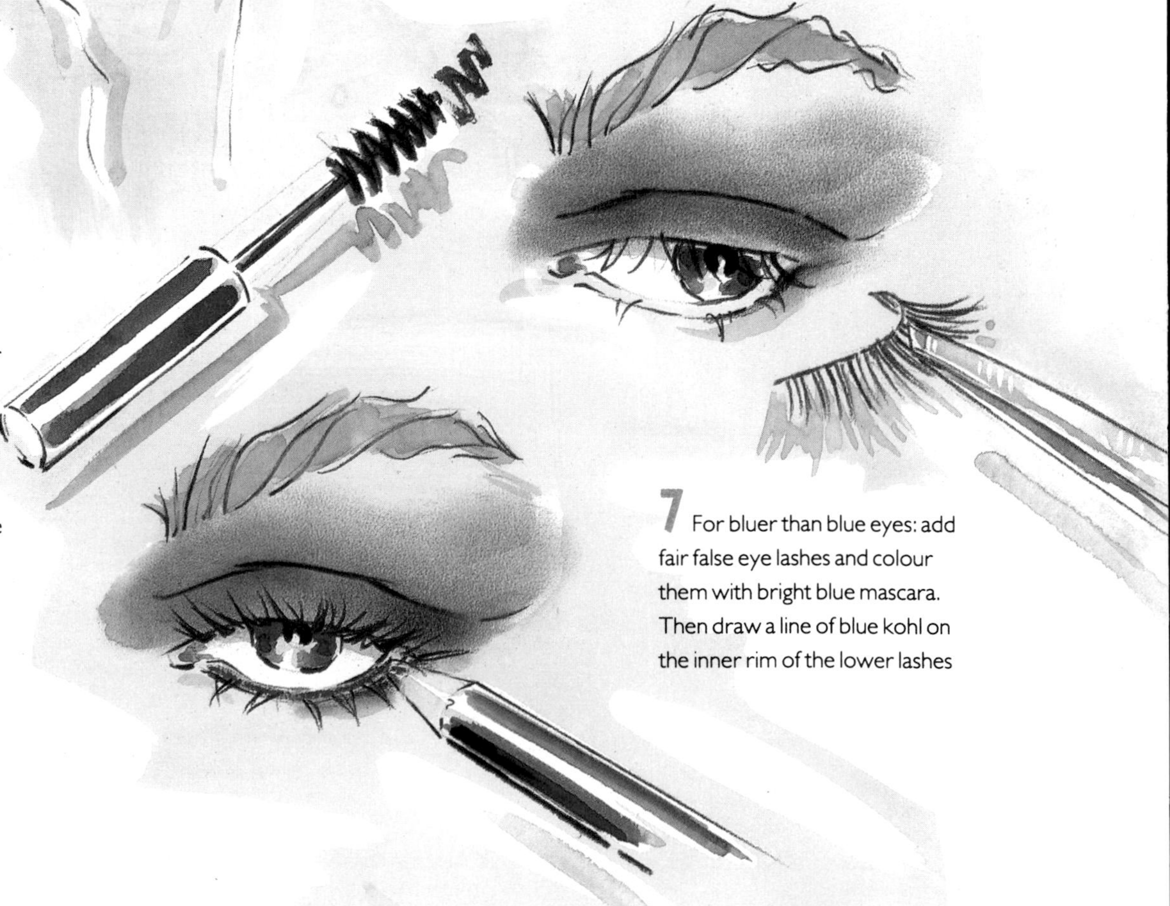

7 For bluer than blue eyes: add fair false eye lashes and colour them with bright blue mascara. Then draw a line of blue kohl on the inner rim of the lower lashes

'. . . don't try a 'trick' for the first time on a special occasion'

8 You can look good when your hair doesn't by tying a turban-like scarf around your head. Use a scarf or a scarf-length piece of any fabric that goes with your outfit. Tie it once round your head, wind it into a concealing turban, tucking the loose ends away. Alternatively, tie the ends into a bow or leave them fanning out from the knot as in our drawing

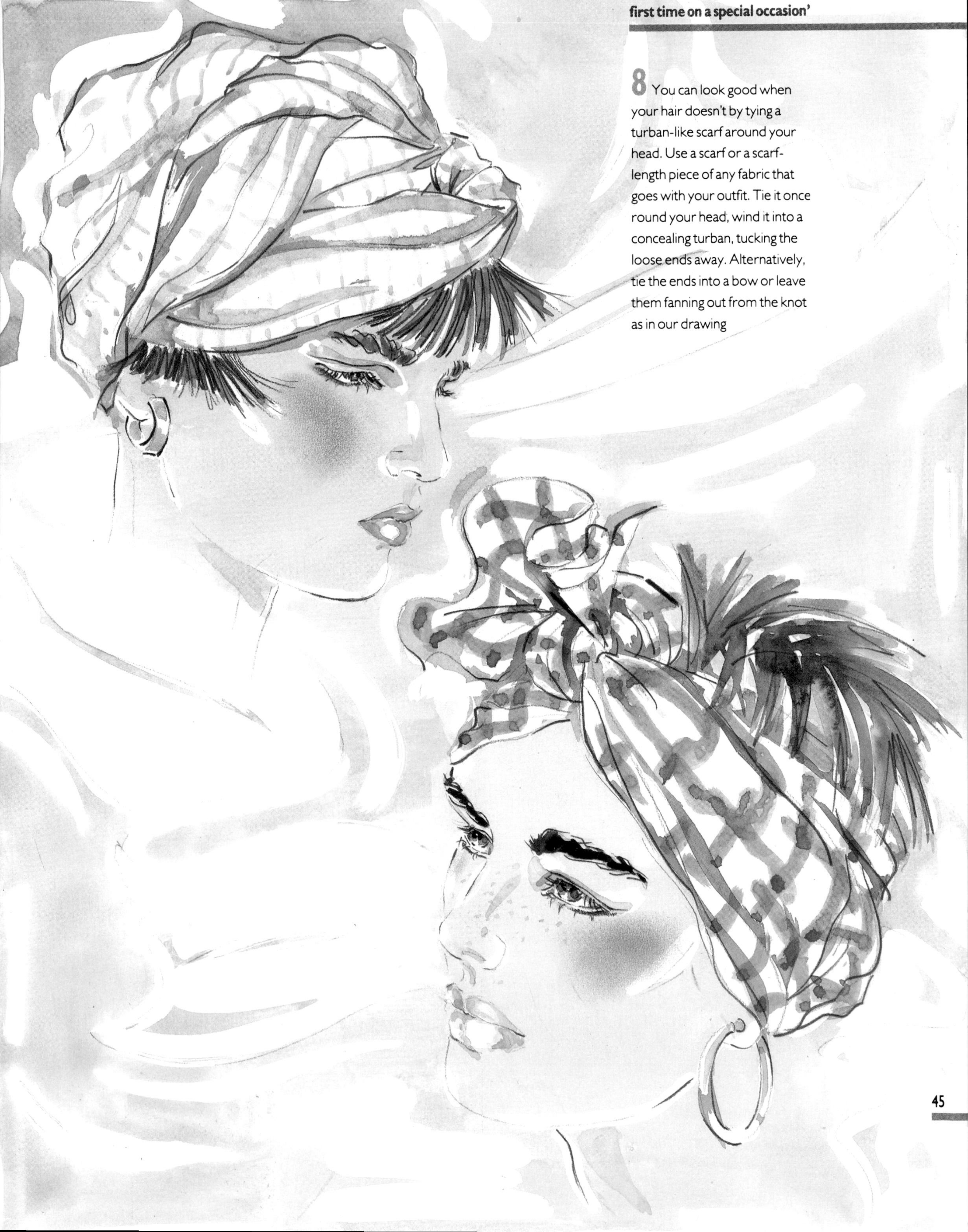

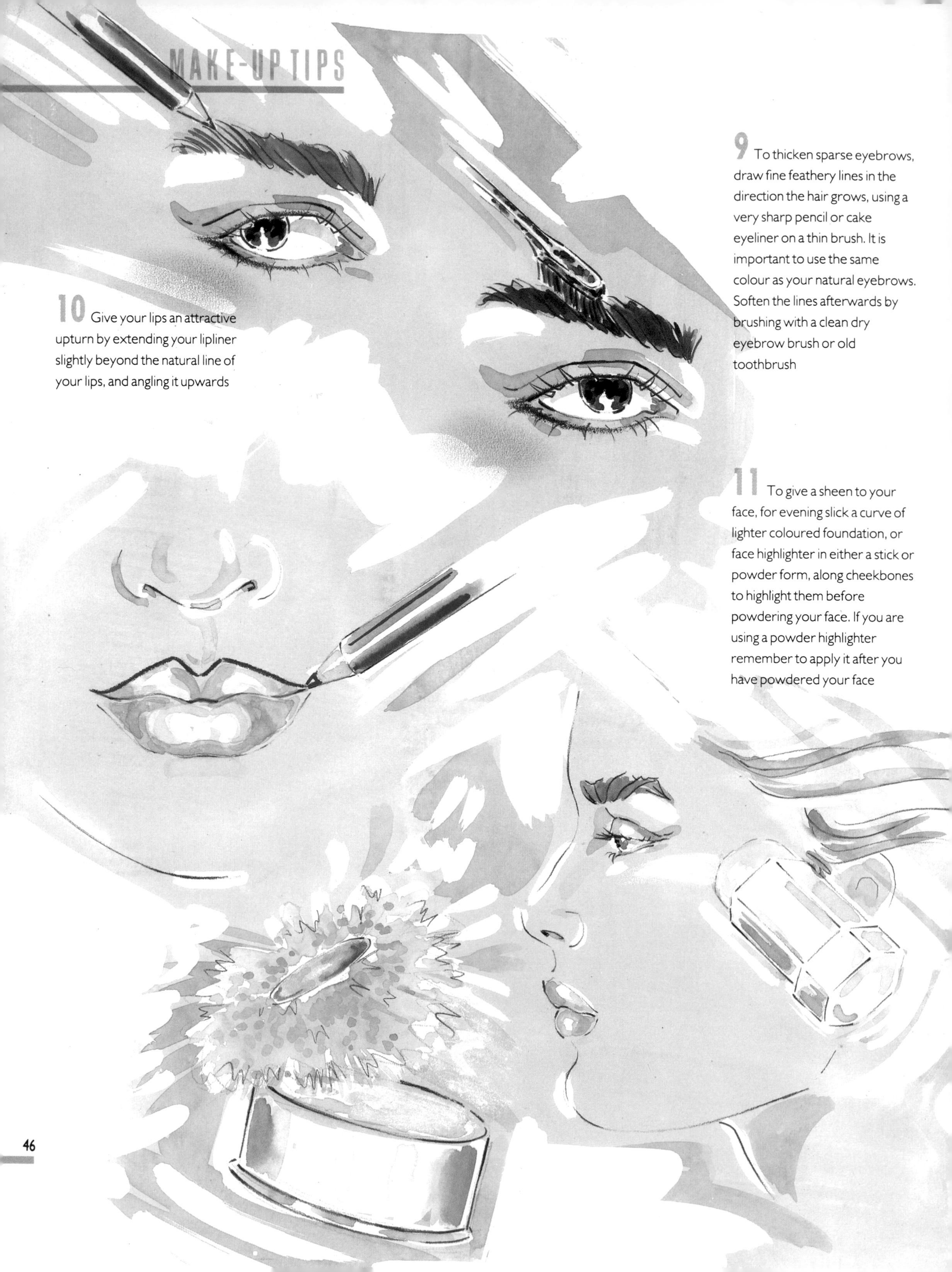

9 To thicken sparse eyebrows, draw fine feathery lines in the direction the hair grows, using a very sharp pencil or cake eyeliner on a thin brush. It is important to use the same colour as your natural eyebrows. Soften the lines afterwards by brushing with a clean dry eyebrow brush or old toothbrush

10 Give your lips an attractive upturn by extending your lipliner slightly beyond the natural line of your lips, and angling it upwards

11 To give a sheen to your face, for evening slick a curve of lighter coloured foundation, or face highlighter in either a stick or powder form, along cheekbones to highlight them before powdering your face. If you are using a powder highlighter remember to apply it after you have powdered your face

'. . . the greatest professional effect relies on. . . patience'

12 To make your eyes look dewy, paint a tiny triangle of highlighter at the inner corner of your eye

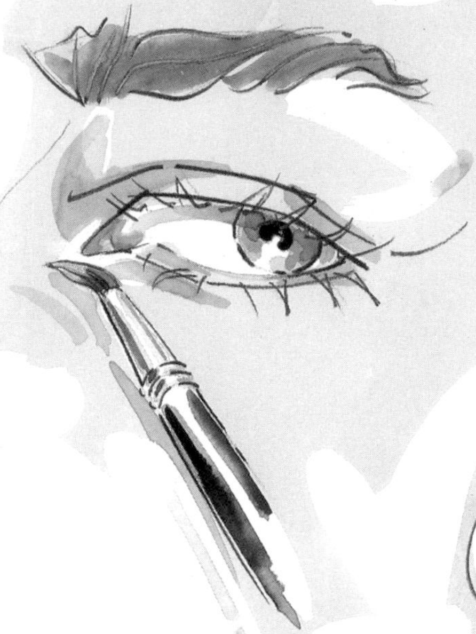

13 For a daytime make-up that makes you look instantly in the pink, use the same pale rose colour on eyes and cheeks as well as your mouth. After applying foundation and concealer, use a pink blusher or pink eyeshadow on your browbone and cheeks. Dust with face powder, then simply add mascara and a matching pink lipstick or lip gloss

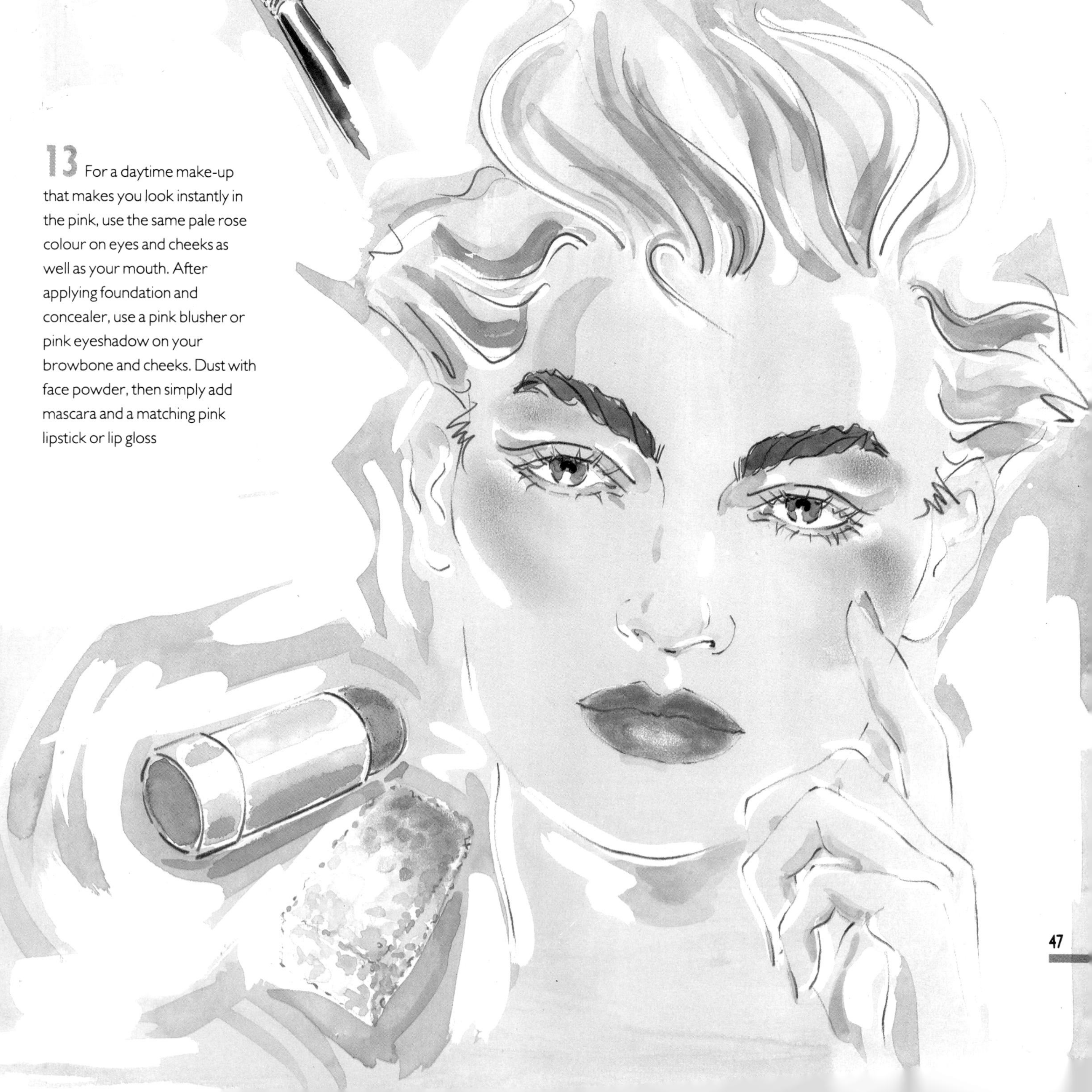

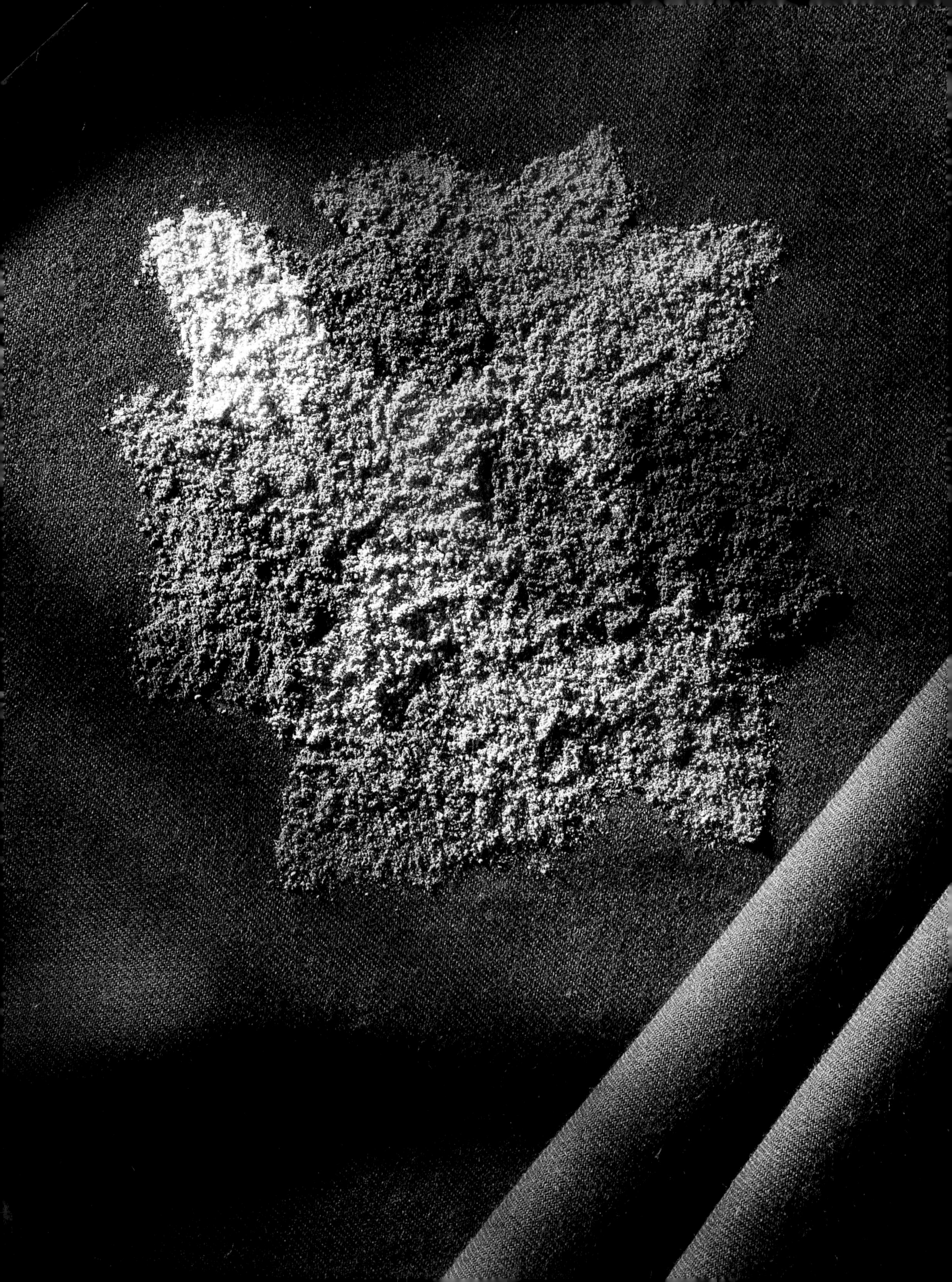

COLOUR COUNSEL

The make-up you wear can be different every day — depending on your mood, the occasion, the colours of your clothes. Your own colouring is the one constant factor, and in the past women dared not experiment because of so-called colour rules. But there is no colour that you cannot wear on your face or clothes, whatever your natural colouring. The models on the following pages represent the main types: blonde, 'mouse', redhead, dark haired and black girl, and they have been dressed and made-up to flout all the old-fashioned rules and show how sensational colour anarchy is. The aim is to give you freedom to try whatever it is you think will look good on you — not to copy exactly any of the make-ups on the following pages, but to spark off ideas for a make-up that is individually yours.

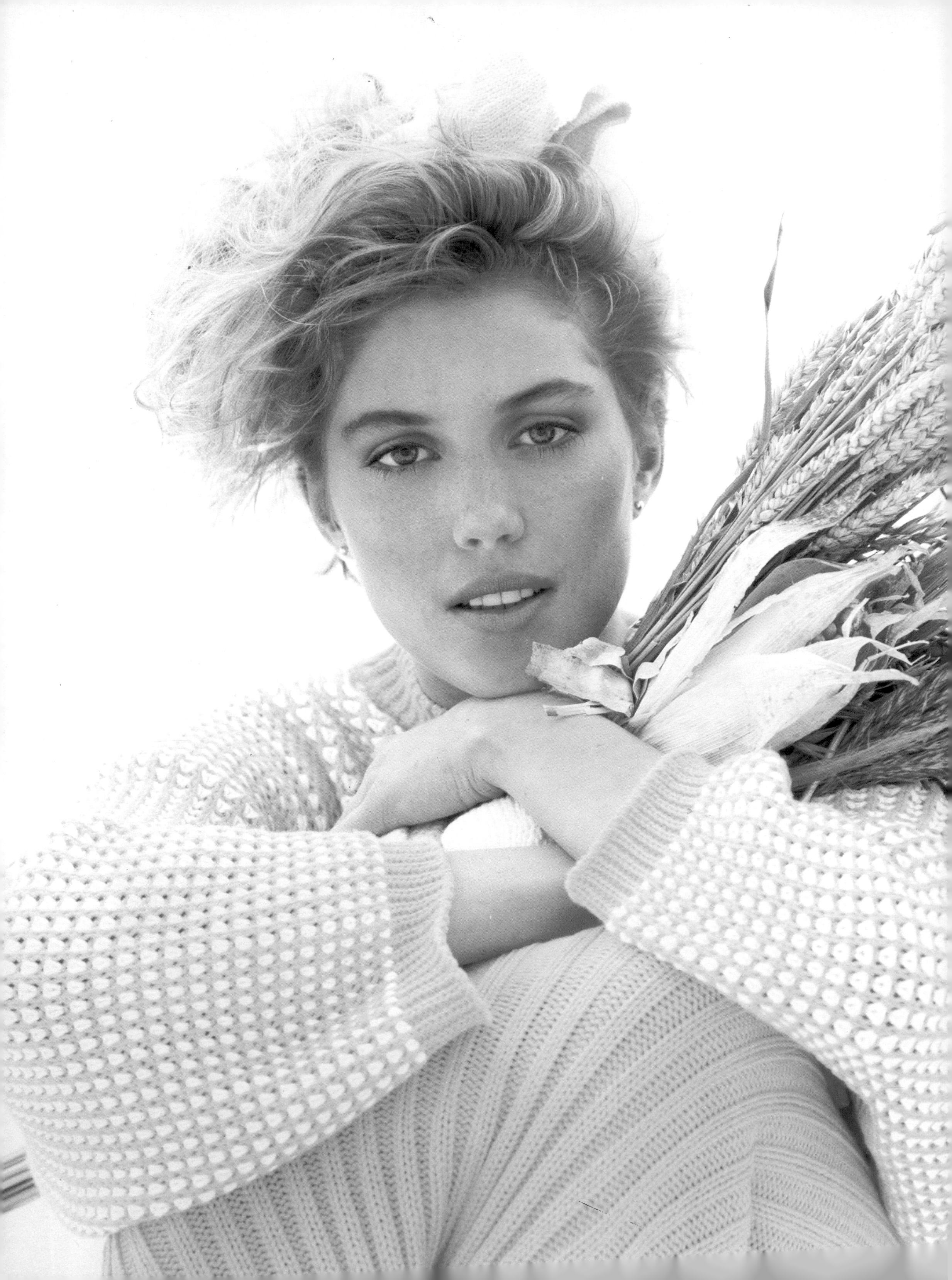

BARELY YELLOW

Yellow is spring and summer, a vibrant, happy colour blondes are often told not to wear. But the right yellow looks sensational. Strong and warm, lifted by touches of pure white, it gives you a sunny, natural, glowing look.

Insipid yellows tinged with lime are not for you. They deprive your complexion of colour, making you look sallow and your hair seem dingy.

But this clear bright yellow enhances all the best things about your colouring – hair looks blonder, and the contrast with sapphire blue eyes is stunning.

The country look is simple and uncluttered: no jewellery, subtly different make-up that gives a fresh glow to your face, and tousled hair caught up with a casually tied piece of matching fabric.

'Tousled hair works best if the style is full. To achieve this effect, I worked gel into the hair and set the front in stand-up pin curls, with large rollers around the sides and back. It was then sprayed with water and dried. After removing the rollers I worked through the hair with my fingers until the curls looked softly untidy.' **J F**

Clothes: Joseph Tricot ·

TECHNICAL TIPS

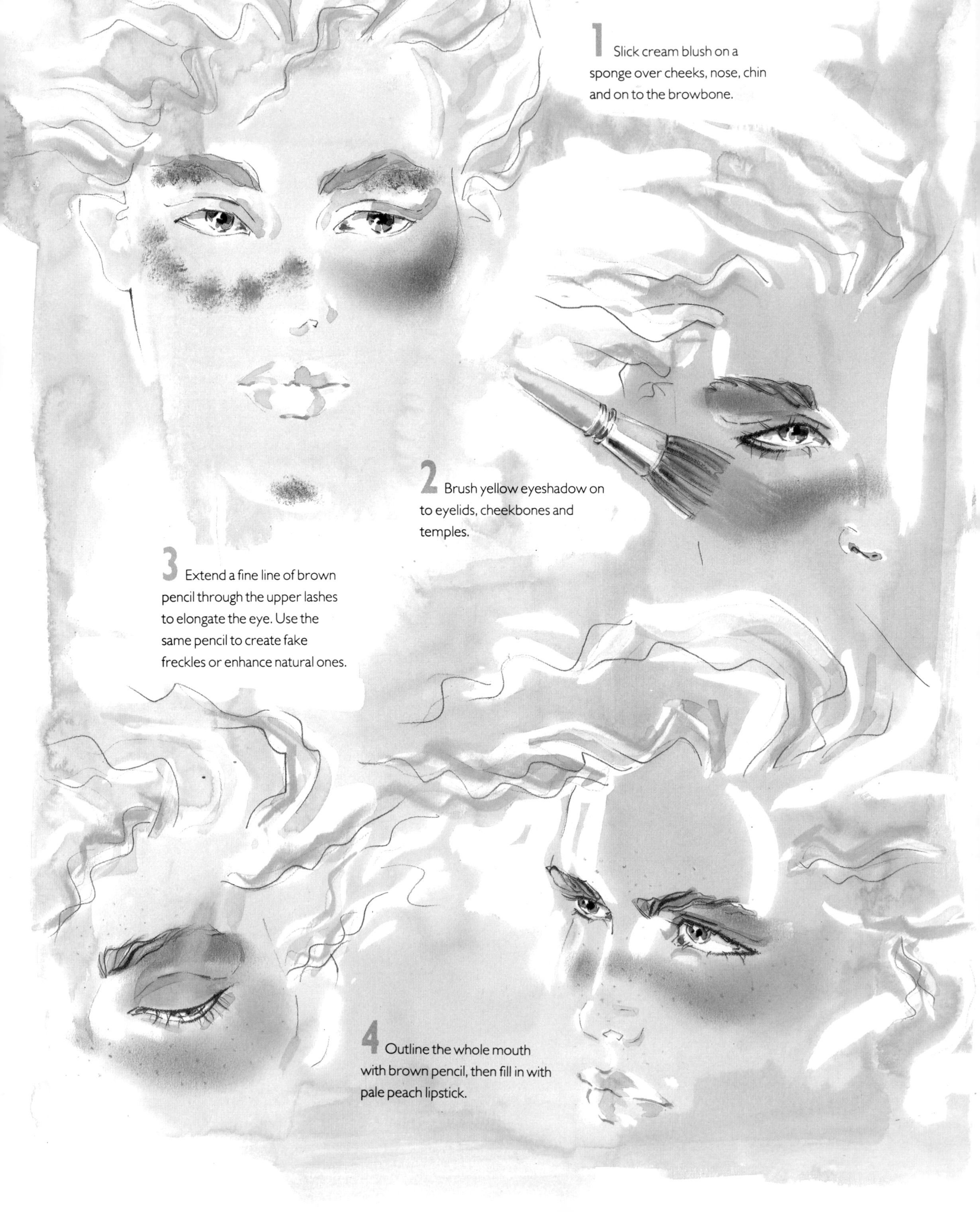

1 Slick cream blush on a sponge over cheeks, nose, chin and on to the browbone.

2 Brush yellow eyeshadow on to eyelids, cheekbones and temples.

3 Extend a fine line of brown pencil through the upper lashes to elongate the eye. Use the same pencil to create fake freckles or enhance natural ones.

4 Outline the whole mouth with brown pencil, then fill in with pale peach lipstick.

BARELY YELLOW

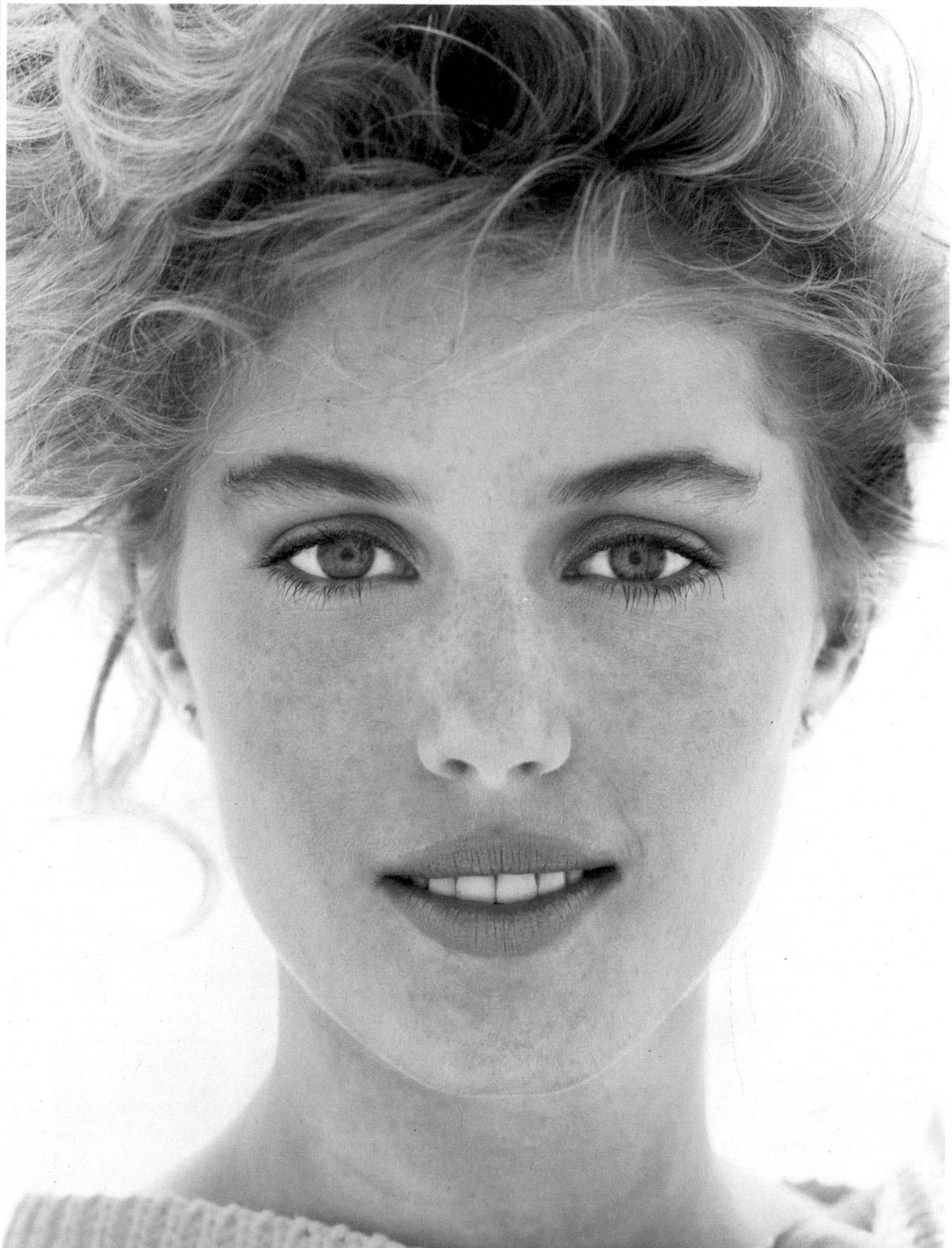

The fresh, outdoor look was achieved by using a tan-tinted gel base for the look of tanned skin. Cream blush on a sponge was slicked over cheeks, nose, chin and on to the brow bone to give a glow. The effect was softened by a light dusting with transparent powder. Yellow eyeshadow was used to tie together the sunny look – on eyelids, cheekbones and temples. Fake freckles were created and natural ones deepened with a twist of brown pencil. A fine brown pencil line through the upper lashes was extended to elongate the eye, and at the outer corner of the lower lashes defined the shape. Brown mascara kept the lashes natural-looking. Peach powder blusher was fluffed on the cheeks with a soft brush. The top lip was outlined with brown, as was the lower lip – then the entire mouth was filled in lightly with pale peach lipstick.

WILD ROSE

Pink is versatile. From baby-pink to dusty old rose, the range of shades and tones gives the lie to the out-dated rule that blondes should avoid it. Baby pinks are not a good choice, but this sexy, sophisticated evening suit in dull pink and smoky lilac shows that pink need never again be considered merely pretty-pretty or girly. Pale pink *can* make blondes look washed-out and insipid, but the stronger and more off-beat shades are very flattering.

The subtle, understated colours of the outfit provide a perfect background for an evening make-up of terrific impact: pale – but very, very interesting. Skin so white it's luminescent; eye colour delicate but clear with a touch of fantasy in the matching eyebrows and eyelashes; and the bold come-hither mouth with its gleaming bright lipstick.

'This hairstyle is wild, but the hair is shining. Setting lotion was worked into the roots, which were lifted with brush and hair-dryer to give maximum volume. The ends were straightened with tongs. Then with hair wax rubbed into the hands I arranged the hair into a gleaming, shaggy mane, using my hands and a comb.' **J F**

Clothes: Joseph pour la Maison · Earrings: Butler & Wilson · Brooch: Monty Don ·

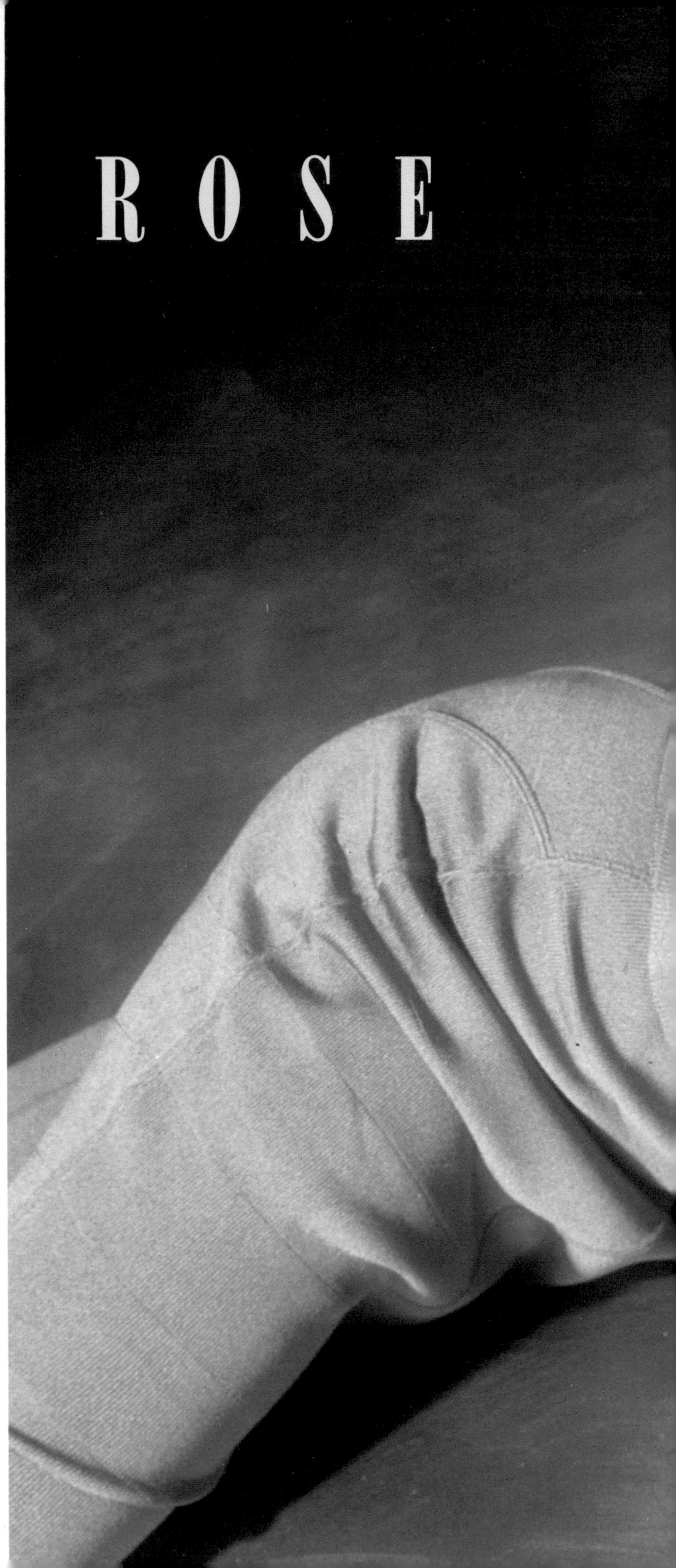

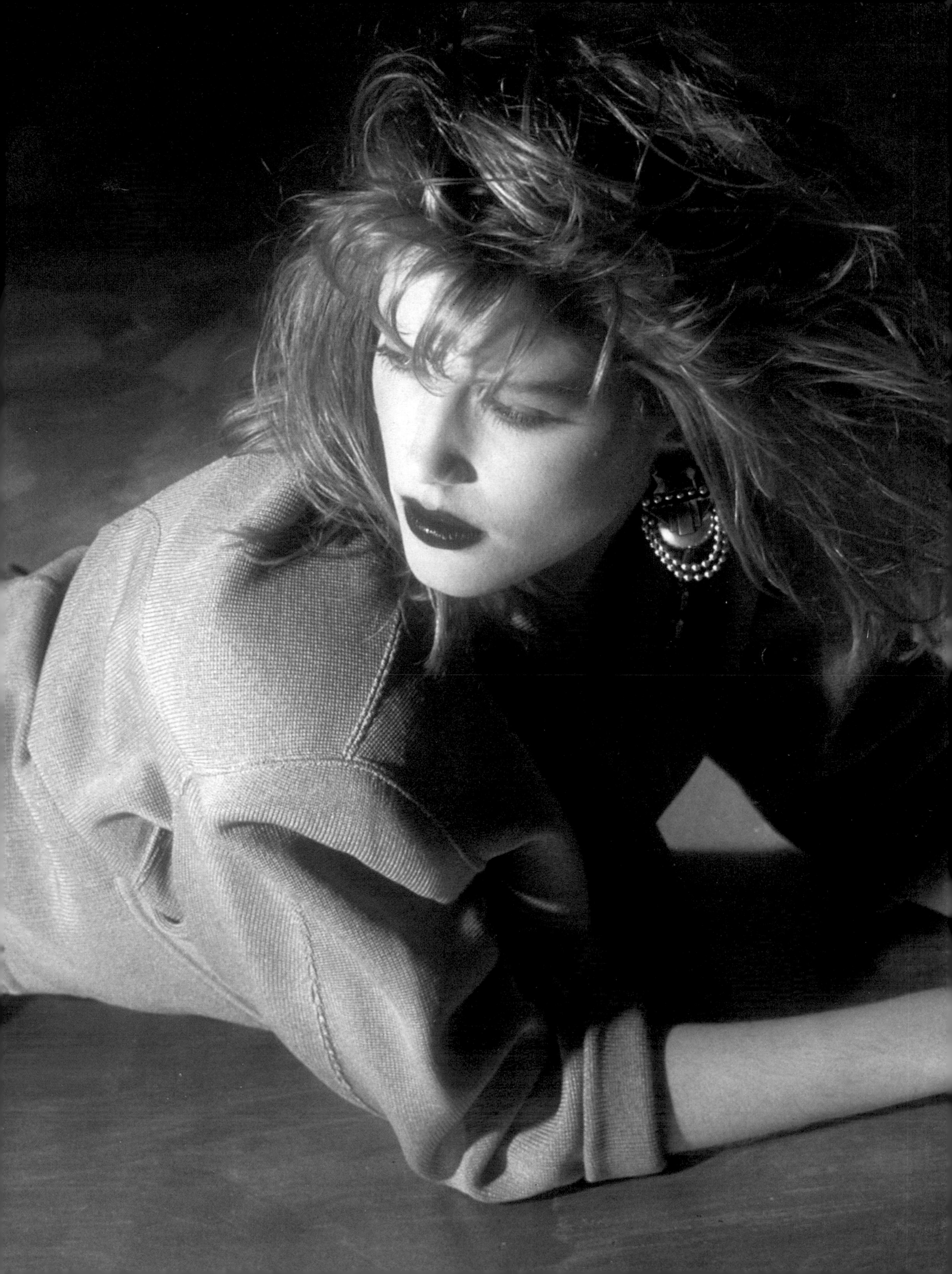

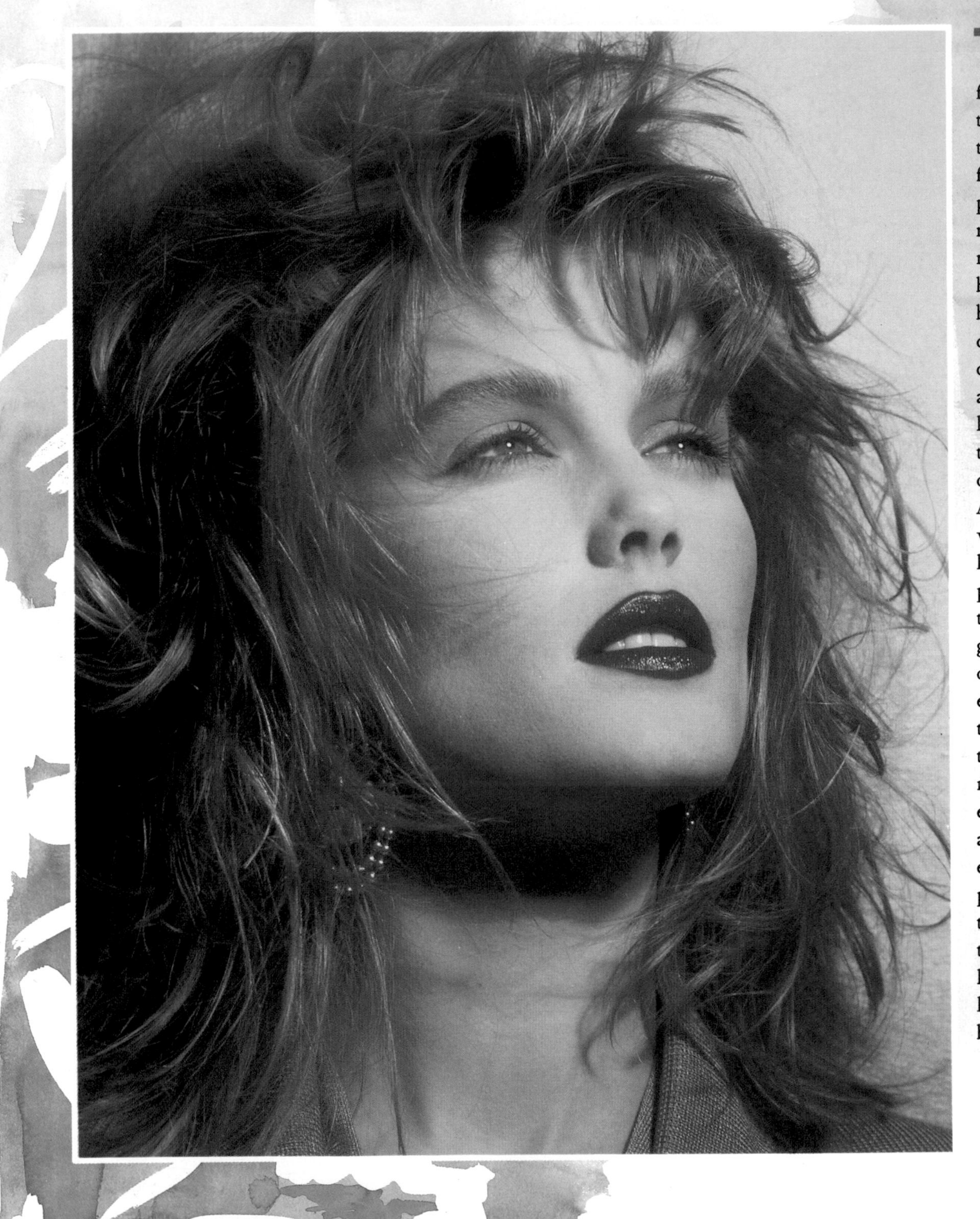

The luminous look needs the palest foundation set with a transparent powder. For the cheeks I mixed white face powder with a bright pink blusher to make it not only paler but also more luminous, and brushed a little over the browbones too. I applied dusky pink eyeshadow all over the upper eyelid, and then blended lavender grey shadow in the crease and on the outer edge of the eyelids. A fine line of plum pencil was used to define the lower eyelid. Pink pearlized highlighter on top of the shadow adds gleam. Lilac mascara co-ordinates the lashes and eyebrows (brushed on to the brows with an old toothbrush). A little mascara on a thin eyeliner brush painted along the top of the eyelashes near the root picks up any eyeshadow that has dropped on to them. Bright fuchsia lipstick completes the look. Apply it with a lip brush for a clean edge.

TECHNICAL TIPS

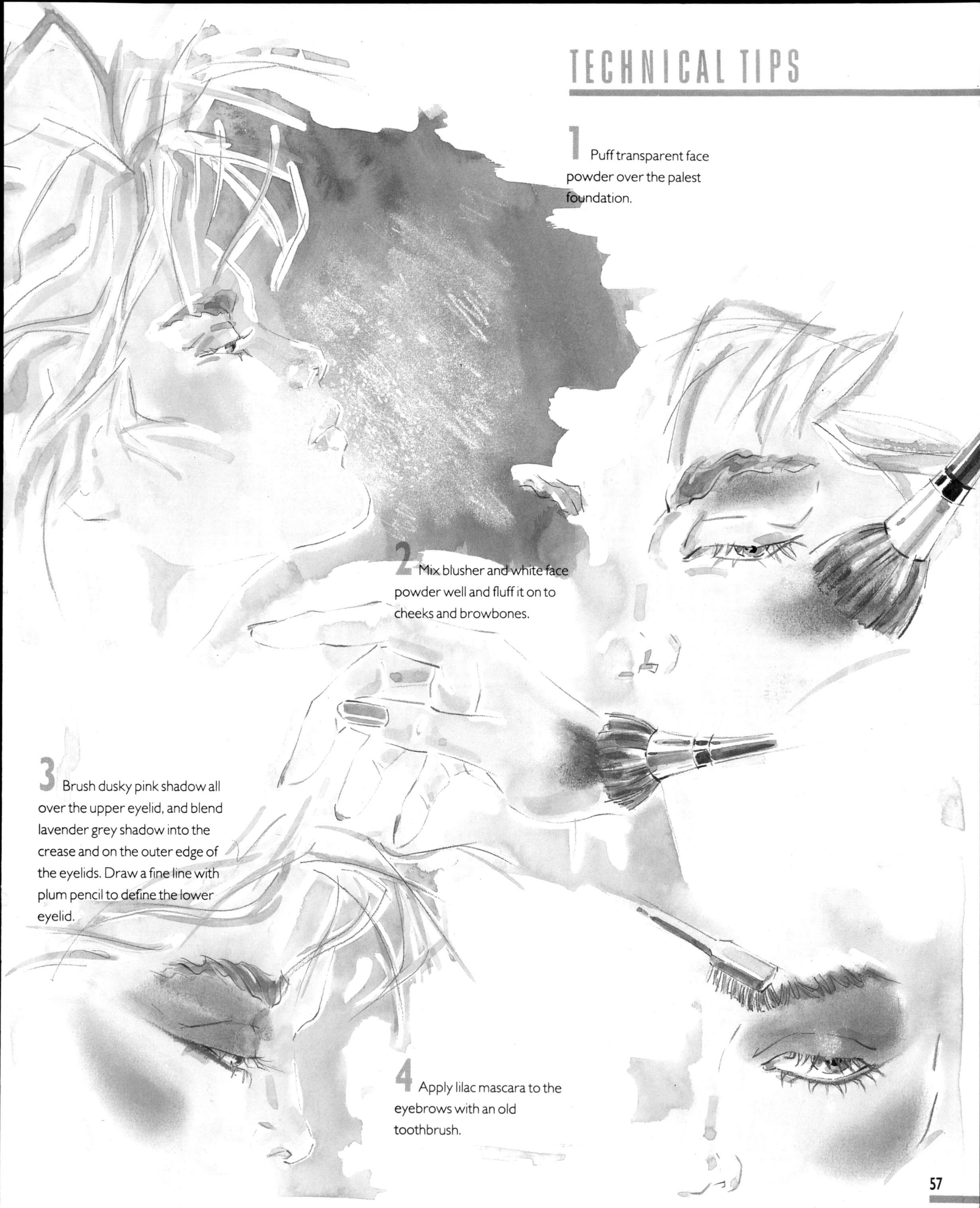

1 Puff transparent face powder over the palest foundation.

2 Mix blusher and white face powder well and fluff it on to cheeks and browbones.

3 Brush dusky pink shadow all over the upper eyelid, and blend lavender grey shadow into the crease and on the outer edge of the eyelids. Draw a fine line with plum pencil to define the lower eyelid.

4 Apply lilac mascara to the eyebrows with an old toothbrush.

Plum has dignity. This sleekly tailored day dress, teamed with a casually cut purple jacket, is proof — if you need it — that blonde doesn't have to mean dizzy. When it comes to cool elegance, blondes have got what it takes — your golden-girl colouring turns so many heads that you can afford to wear the most subtle and understated colour schemes.

A working-girl's make-up needs to be strong, though not heavy or dark, and simple to apply first thing in the morning — like this one. It must make you look good without being too startling.

A clear pink lipstick, witty earrings, and a bold brooch combine to add the finishing touch.

'Hair can look tidy and business-like without being prim and unfeminine. Here it is smoothed into a neat French pleat. A light coating of hair wax or hairspray on your hands makes odd flyaway ends easy to tidy into place. The asymmetric fringe adds sexiness to a classic style.' **J F**

Dress: Maxfield Parrish · Jacket: John McIntyre · Brooch: Monty Don · Earrings: Gary Wright & Sheila Teague ·

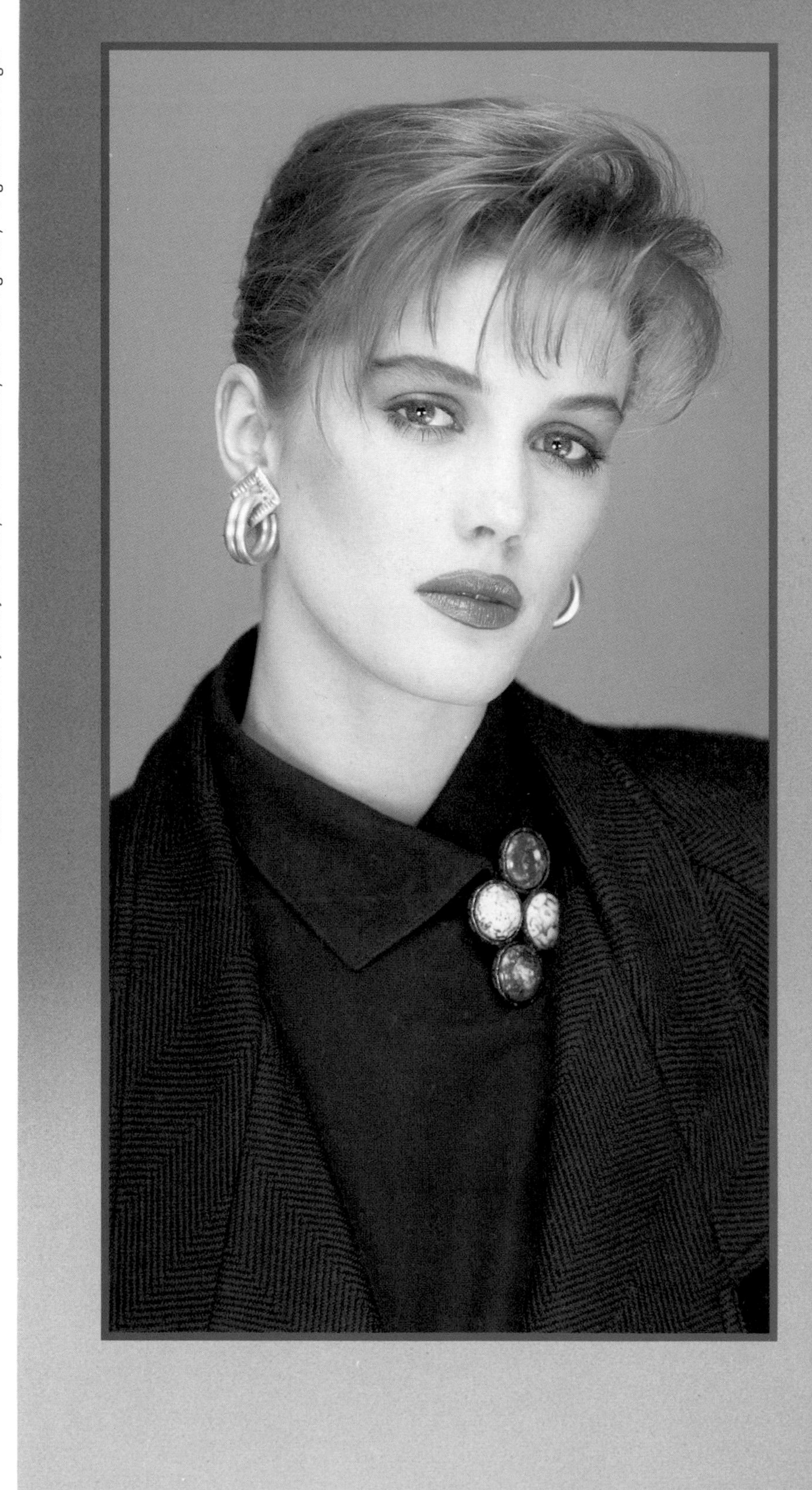

PLUM CRAZY

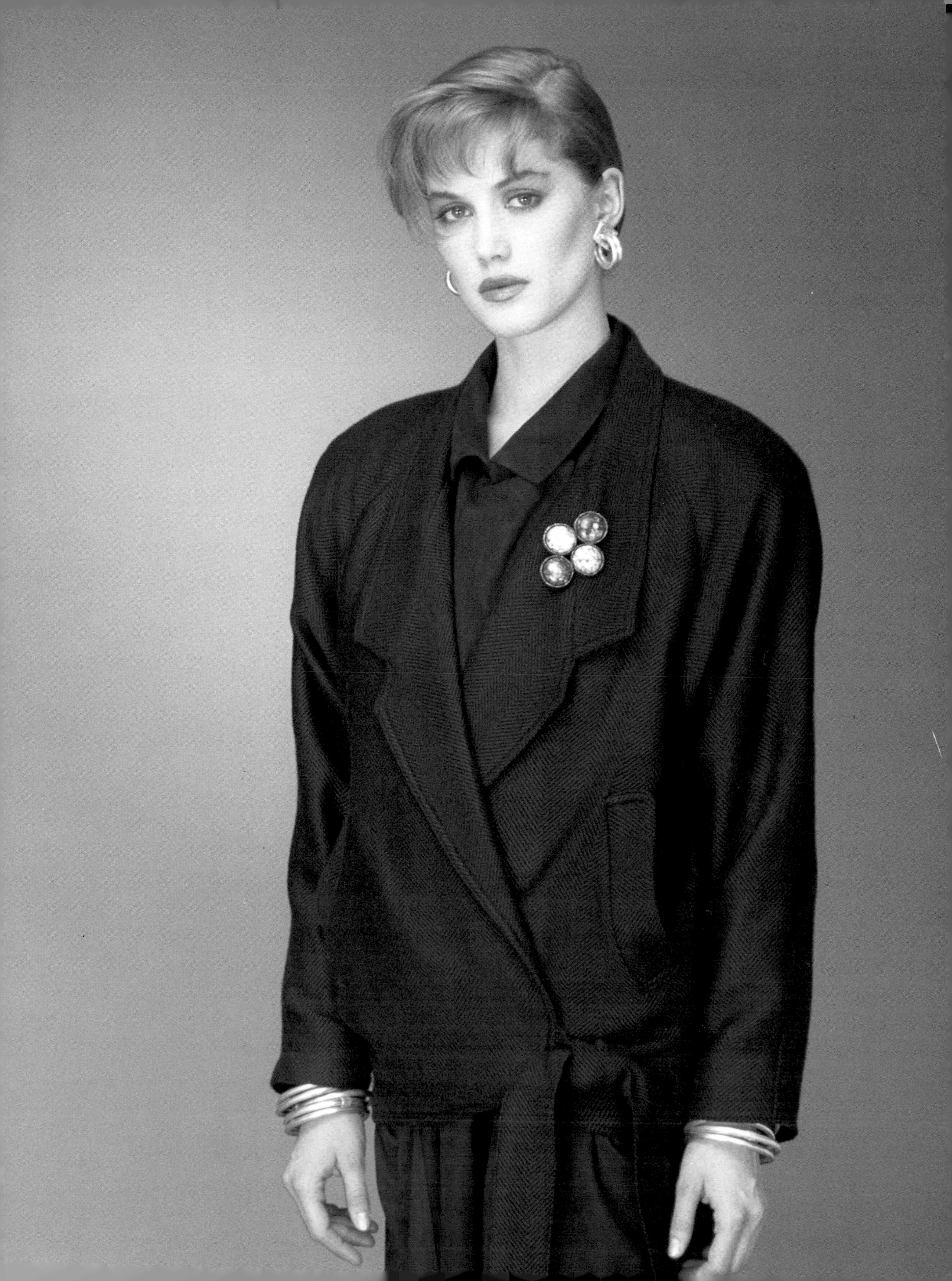

The working woman's make-up starts with foundation that matches skin tone, set with a light dusting of powder. I used smoky grey shadow, worked in with a brush over the entire eyelid. It is more concentrated in the crease, brushed out to its lightest on the browbone, with a smudge blended under the lower lashes. The eyeliner is a powder shadow of the exact plum shade of the dress. Mixed with water it becomes a good cake eyeliner and can be painted on with a fine brush. Pink blusher is used to highlight below the brow, as well as on the cheeks. The eyes are finished with dark brown mascara. A few fine lines pencilled through the eyebrows makes them look thicker. With well-defined eyes the lips can be lighter — a clear pink outlined with a pinky brown pencil for definition.

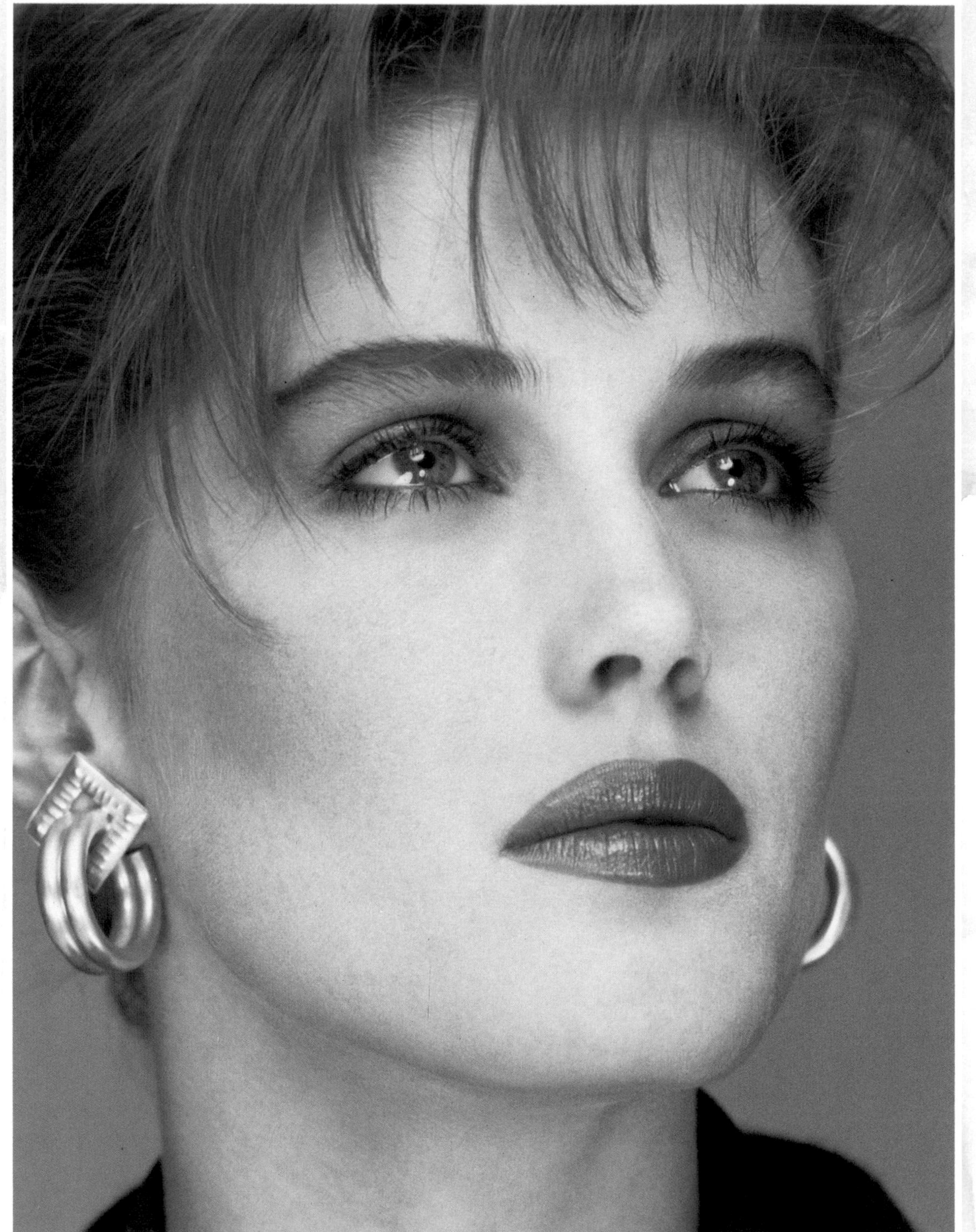

1 Work smoky grey eyeshadow with a brush over the entire upper eyelid, and smudge it under the lower lashes.

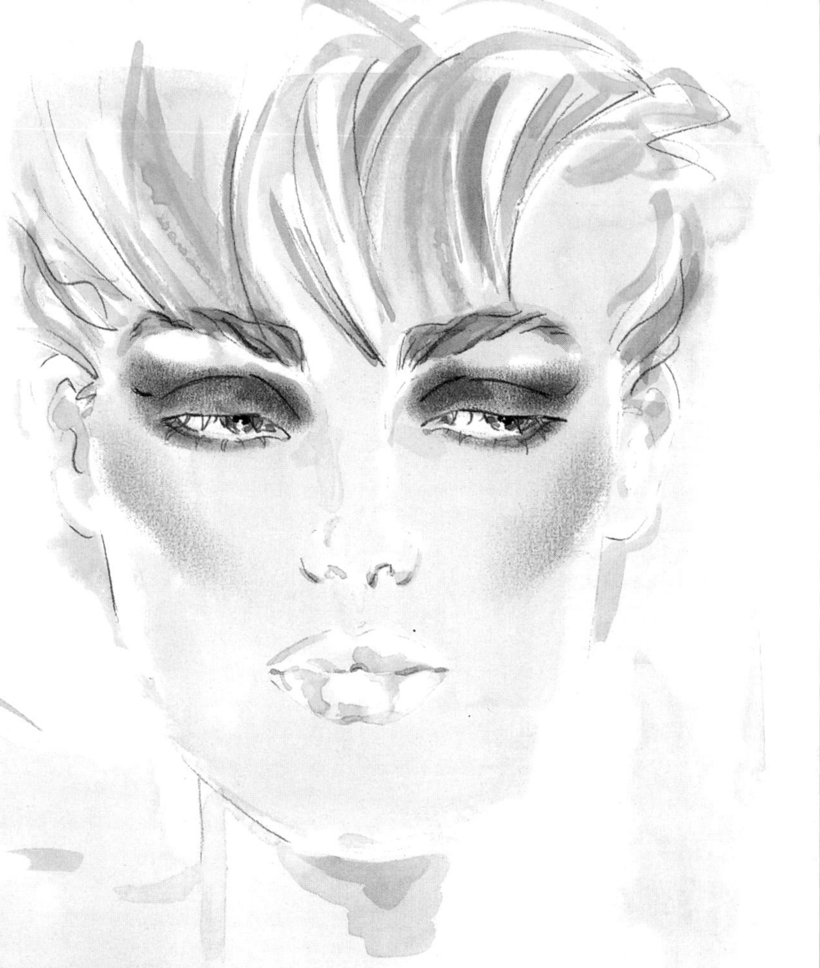

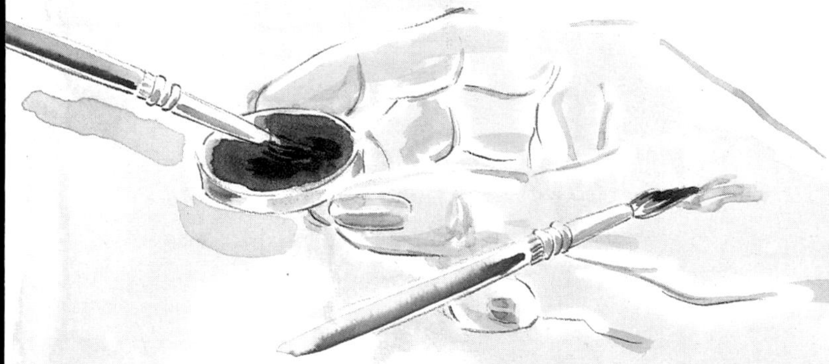

2 Plum eyeshadow mixed with water becomes a good cake eyeliner.

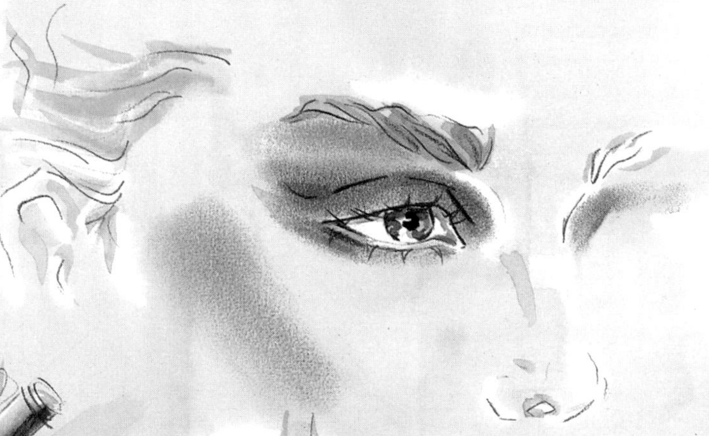

3 Highlight the brow, as well as the cheeks, with pink blusher.

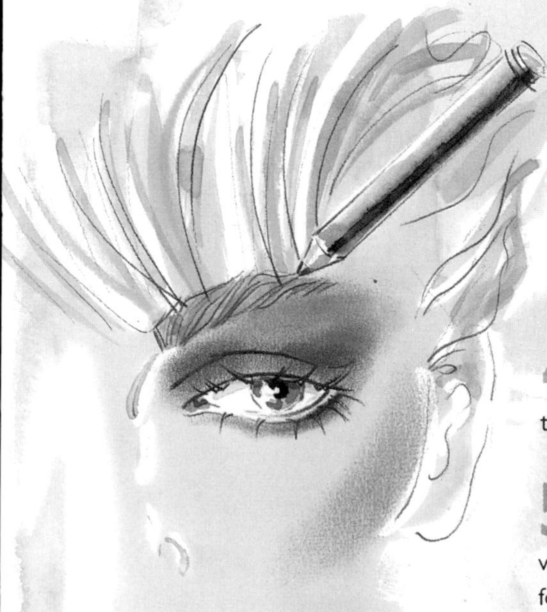

4 Pencil a few fine lines through the eyebrow.

5 Outline clear pink lips with a pinky brown pencil for definition.

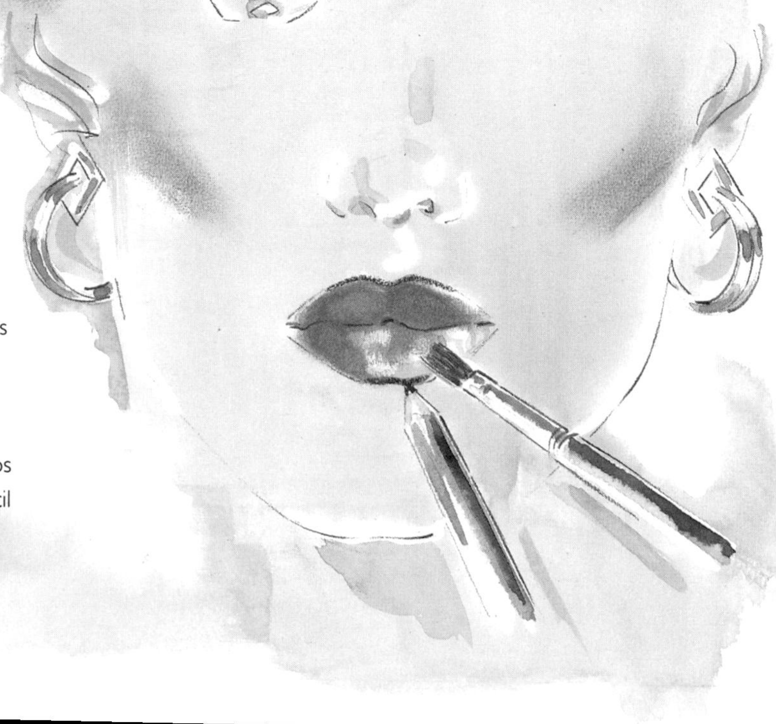

Ivory is the perfect colour for a bride and looks breathtaking. Any girl would feel wonderful wearing a fairy-tale dream of a dress such as this. The fair skin of the English 'mouse' is flattered by this colour, and the reflected ivory highlights give the skin a translucent sheen.

With the flounces, lace and bows of this frock creating the interest, everything else must be simple without being dull. The length of veiling for example, is twirled into a froth, rather than arranged in the traditional way.

Brides are invariably nervous, so make-up needs to be effortless and foolproof. This one really does take only ten minutes from start to finish. A classically pastel bridal theme is given a new look by using yellow and peach, though any two pastel colours – yellow, lavender, pink or blue – used imaginatively together would work.

'This hairstyle is as straightforward to do as the make-up. The hair was dampened and caught back into a ponytail, which was wound round on itself to form a top-knot, then fixed with pins and a hair net. The simple style was finished with a halo of veil.' **J F**

Dress: Tatters

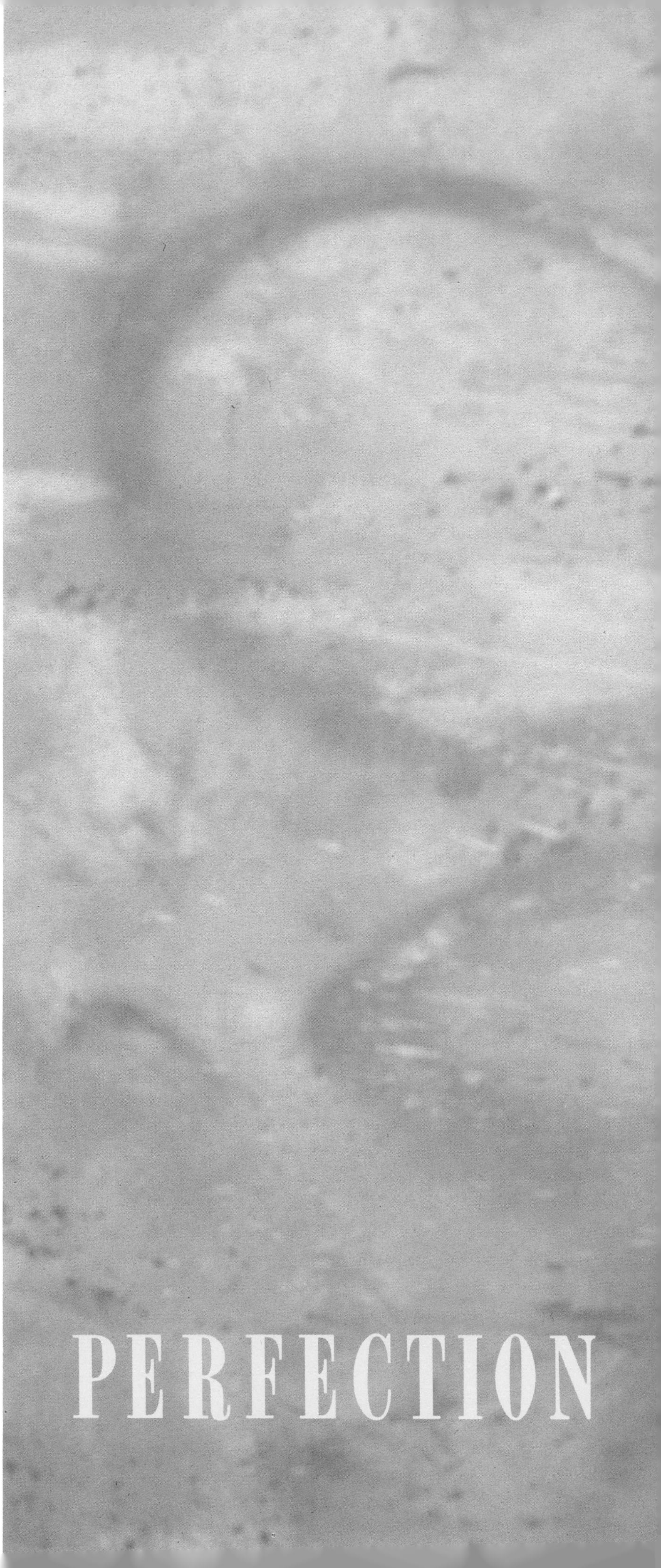

PALE PERFECTION

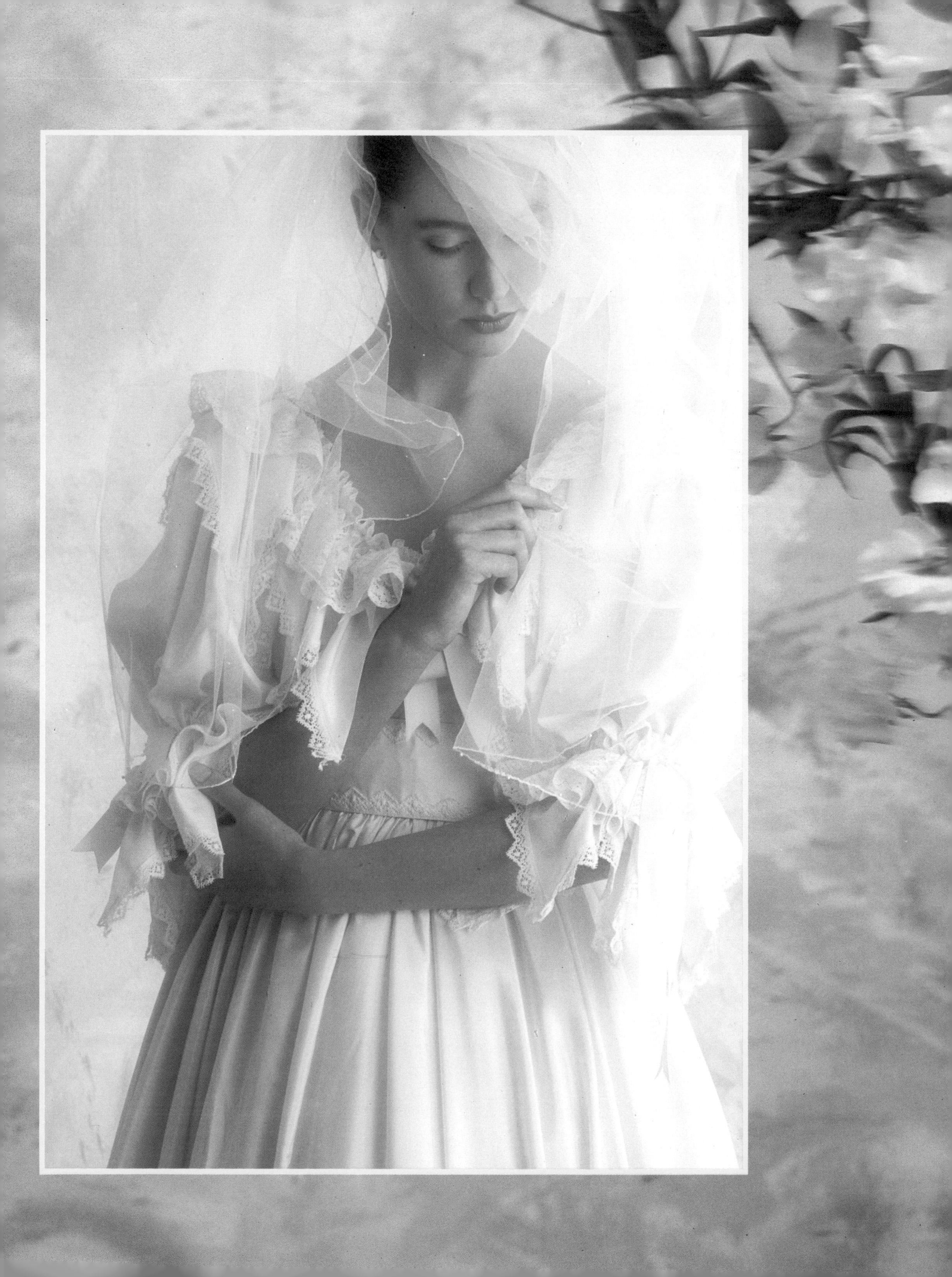

PALE PERFECTION

The bride's make-up starts with a fair, natural-toned foundation, lightly dusted with transparent powder for a porcelain finish. A clear yellow shadow is brushed over the entire eyelid. Strong peach powder shadow is applied just under the eye and at the outer corner of the upper lid, then gently blended out to the side of the eyes, leaving the merest hint of peach. Then I blended the two colours well so that the effect is soft but interesting. Lavender mascara is used on the lashes. Peach blusher is swept over cheekbones and very lightly under the eye. The blusher is powdered over with face powder so the lightest tinge of colour is left. The mouth is made soft and full with peach lipstick applied carefully with a lip brush and well blotted.

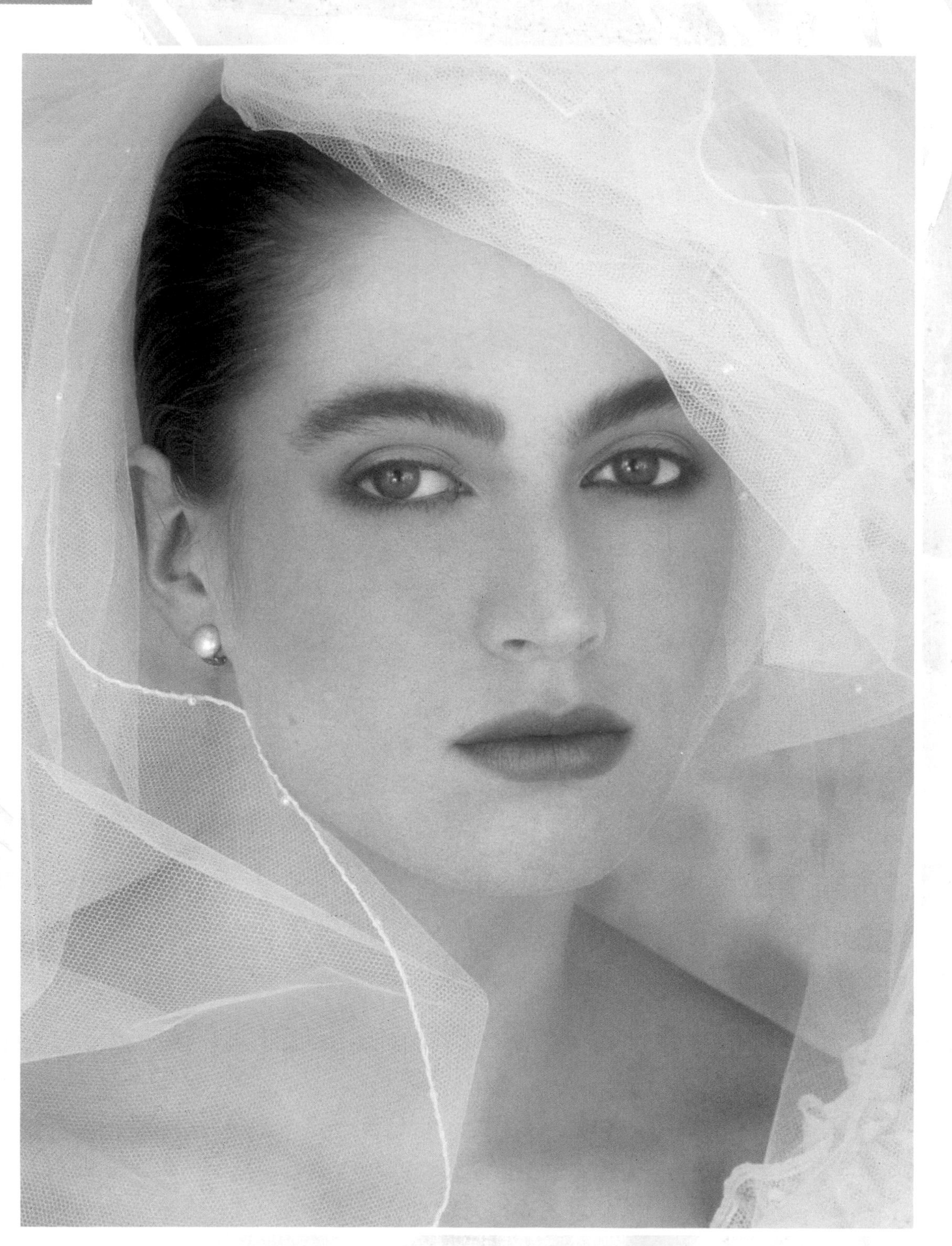

TECHNICAL TIPS

1 Brush clear yellow shadow over the entire eyelid.

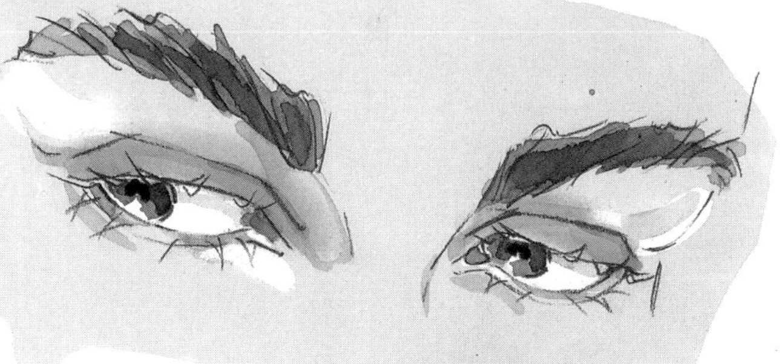

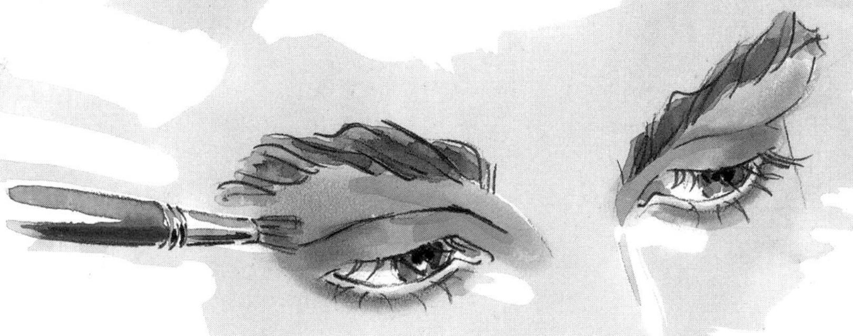

2 Apply peach eyeshadow under the eye and at the outer corner of the upper lid, then blend gently out to the side of the eyes.

3 Sweep peach blusher over the cheekbones and very lightly under the eye.

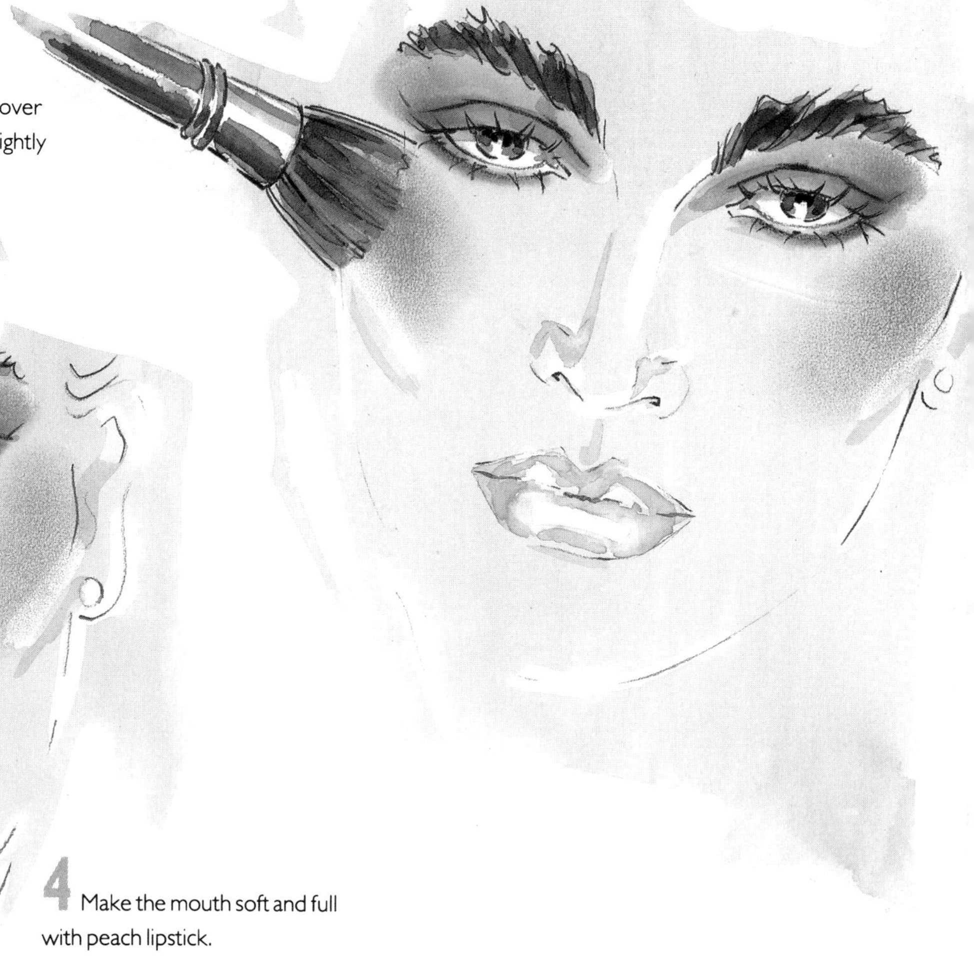

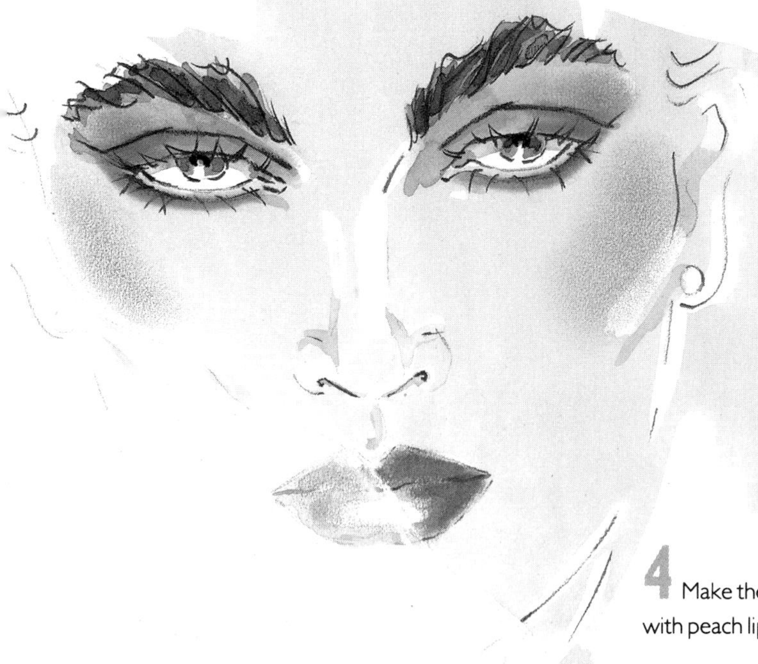

4 Make the mouth soft and full with peach lipstick.

ICED COFFEE

Camel is a classically elegant colour – but a difficult shade to wear if you have pale brown hair and the general colouring to match. 'Mousy' women are usually advised to steer clear of it in case they end up looking dull and monochromatic. But clever dressing and clever make-up can make the cool tones of camel more than simply succeed. They can look quite dramatic against the quiet-toned colouring of the traditional mouse. One secret is to add white to the clothes, either with a T-shirt similar to the one our model is wearing or with white accessories.

The other essential is to add brightness to your face: not necessarily on the cheeks, which can be milky pale, nor with bold eyes, which look good as a smoothly blended mix of honey shades; but with pink on the lips – the only contrasting colour in the entire ensemble.

'For this look, I set Ursula's hair in large rollers following its own natural wave, then brushed it out using the drier, to tame flyaway ends and give a smoothly polished and flawless finish to match the elegance of the clothes.' **J F**

Clothes: Sonia Rykiel at Browns · Shoes: Maud Frizon · Earrings: Butler & Wilson ·

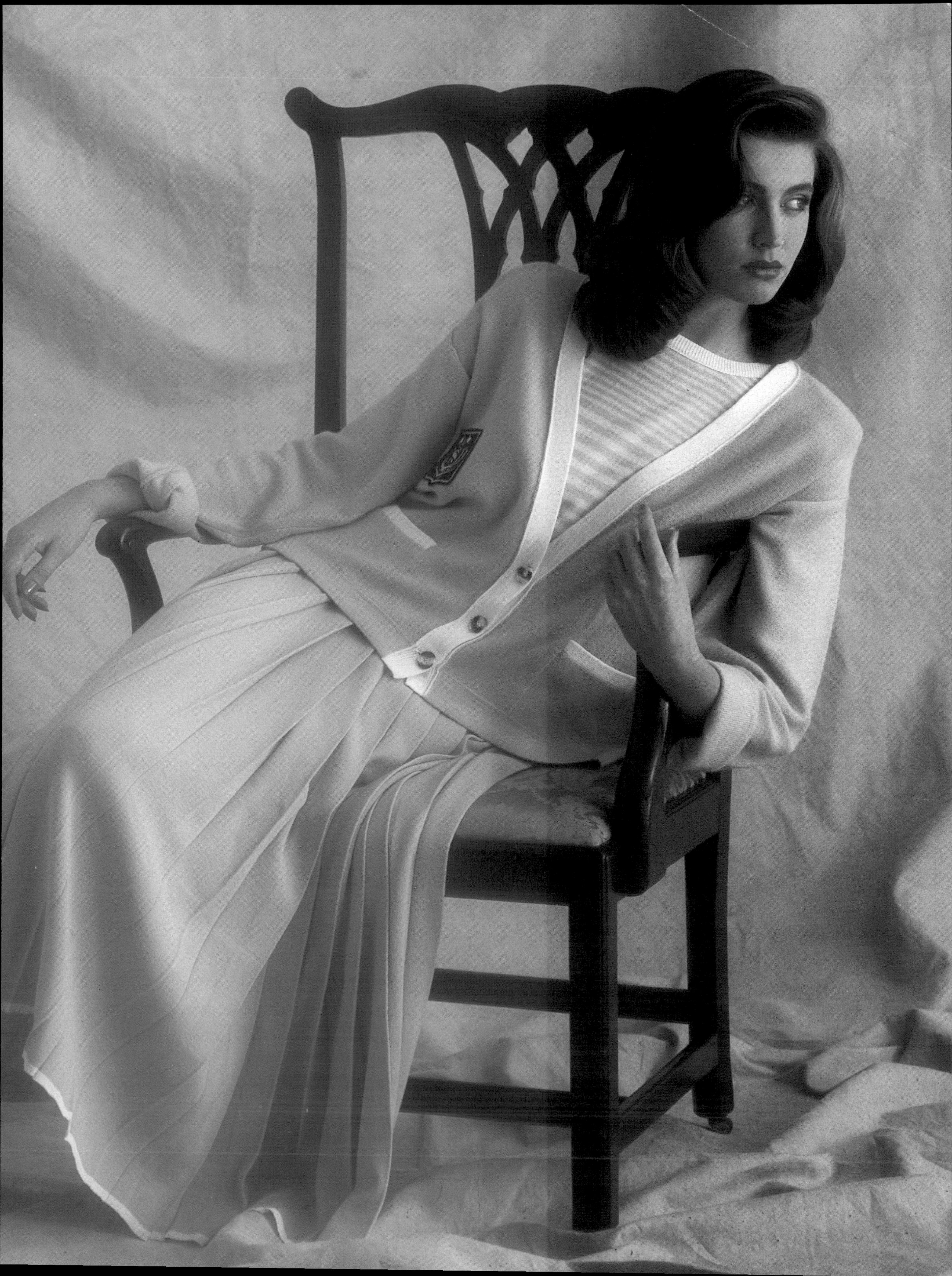

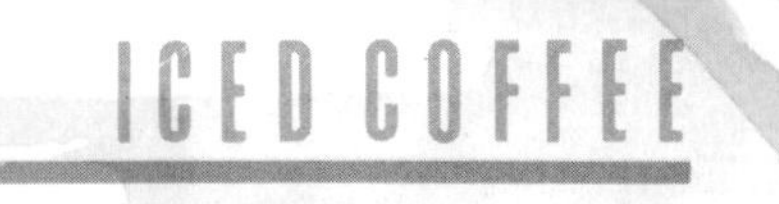

ICED COFFEE

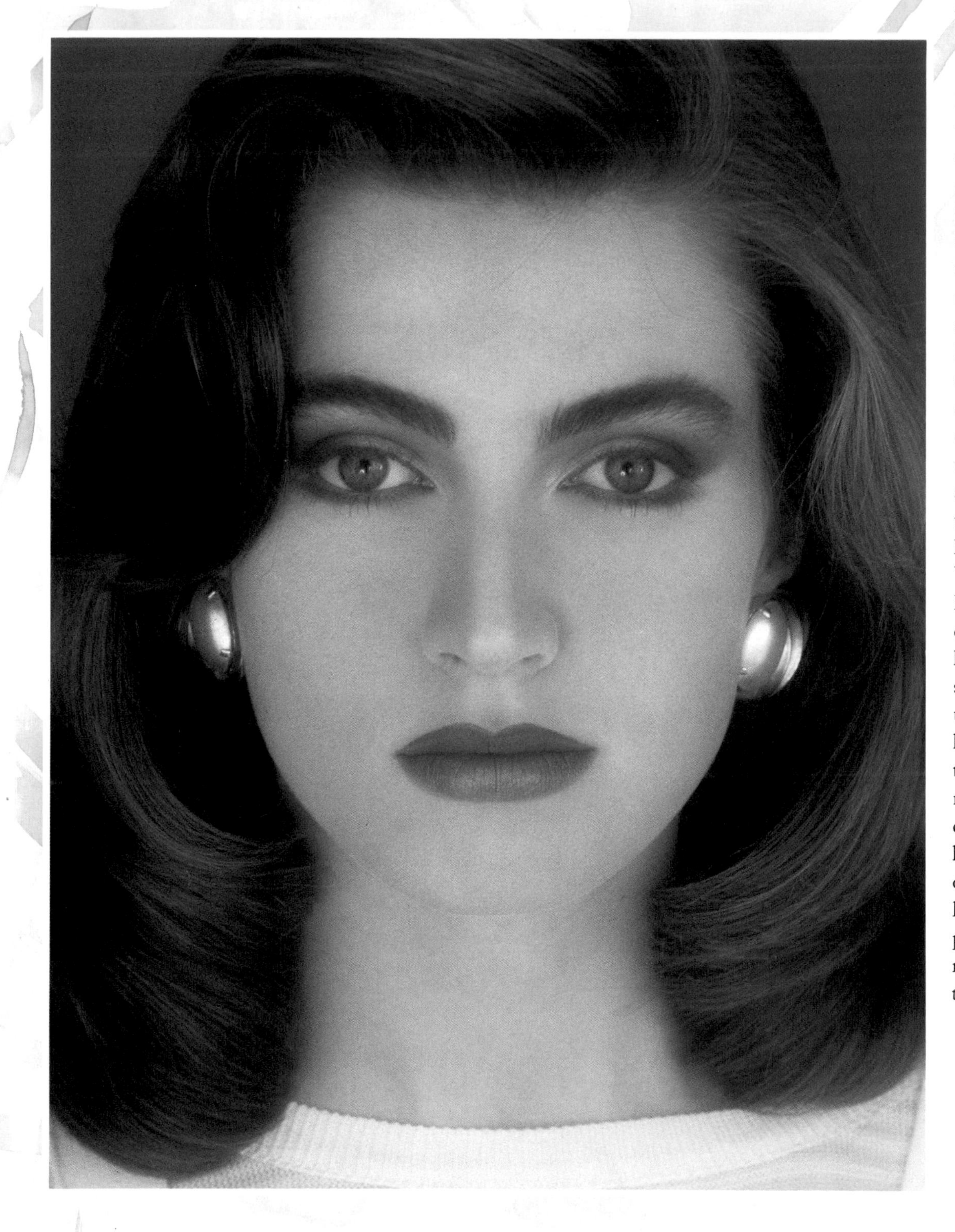

This cool classic look has a pale base, lightly powdered, without any blusher. The eyes are defined by an orangey-brown make-up pencil as soft as a crayon, drawn into the crease of the eyelid, and blended up to the browbone with a brush. I used golden brown powder eyeshadow at the outer corner of the upper eyelid, blending it upwards and outwards and at the sides. A line of the same shadow is blended under the eye. Yellowy-cream highlighter is used as a contrast in the 'V' shape between top and bottom shadows. A little is also used to highlight the brow and the inner half of the upper eyelid. Auburn mascara, which has colour impact without being heavy, is stroked on the lashes. The upper lip is defined with a lip pencil in clear rose, which matches the lipstick used to fill in the whole mouth.

TECHNICAL TIPS

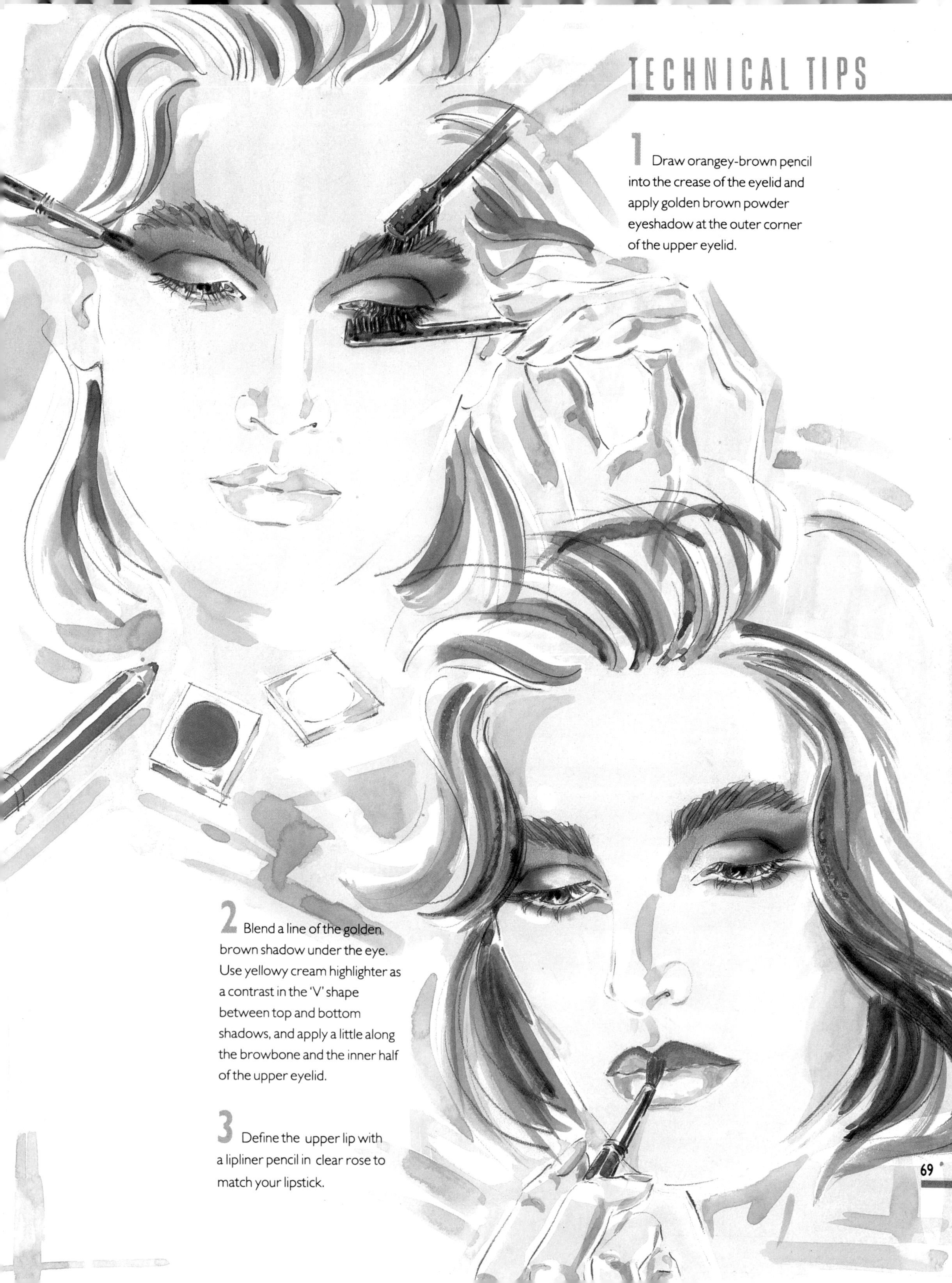

1 Draw orangey-brown pencil into the crease of the eyelid and apply golden brown powder eyeshadow at the outer corner of the upper eyelid.

2 Blend a line of the golden brown shadow under the eye. Use yellowy cream highlighter as a contrast in the 'V' shape between top and bottom shadows, and apply a little along the browbone and the inner half of the upper eyelid.

3 Define the upper lip with a lipliner pencil in clear rose to match your lipstick.

SCARLET LADY

Black is anything you want it to be – elegant, sombre or sexy. With scarlet it marks a metamorphosis from tame mouse to compelling siren.

The clean mannish lines of this suit are as versatile as its colour. With a simple shirt it is a picture of quiet elegance, but the soft drape of this scarf and mellow colours of the jewellery turn the look into something ultra-feminine.

When black is the predominant colour, make-up looks most striking if it is keyed to the accessories. Here the red mouth matches the scarf, and the unusual combination of colours on the eyes was chosen to match the jewellery.

'To turn the hair into a mane of windswept locks, first plenty of mousse was worked through, then it was scrunch-dried with the hands. More body was given by lifting the roots with a comb and directing the drier on to the roots. I drew the hair to one side, secured it with large combs, then backcombed it a little and sprayed it lightly to hold the side-sweep.' **J F**

Suit: Sonia Rykiel at Browns · Scarf: Whistles · Jewellery: Monty Don·

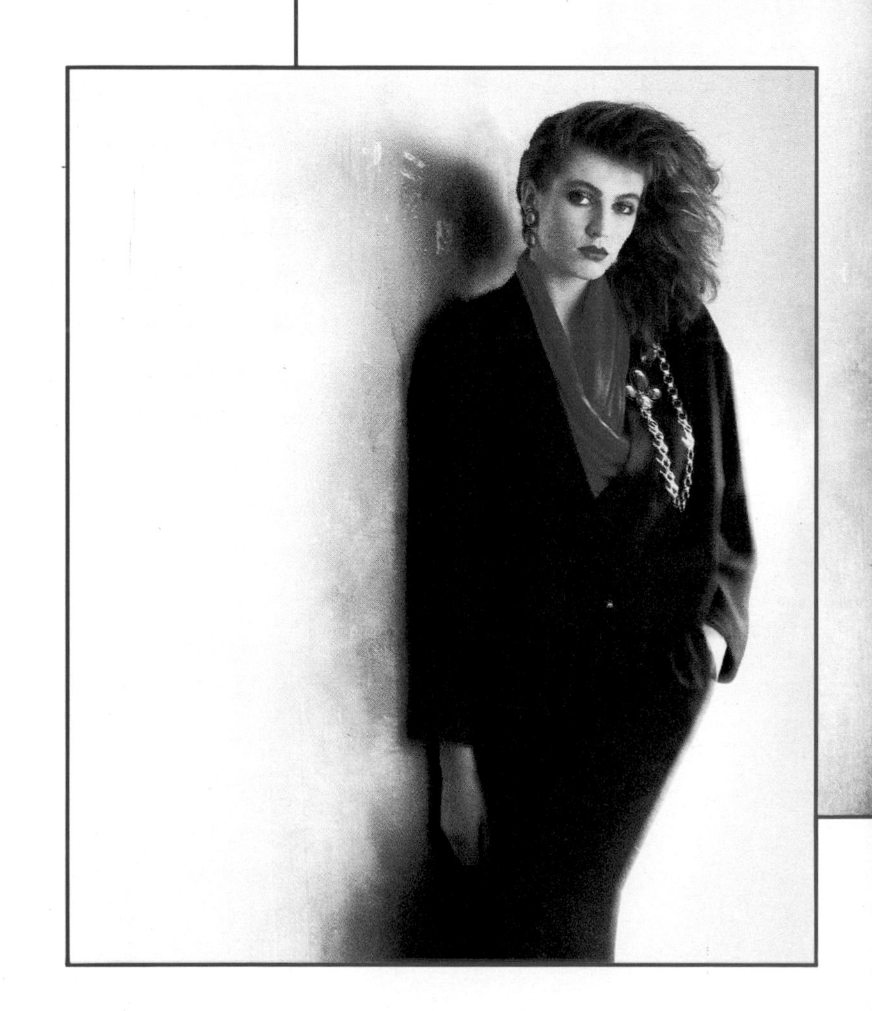

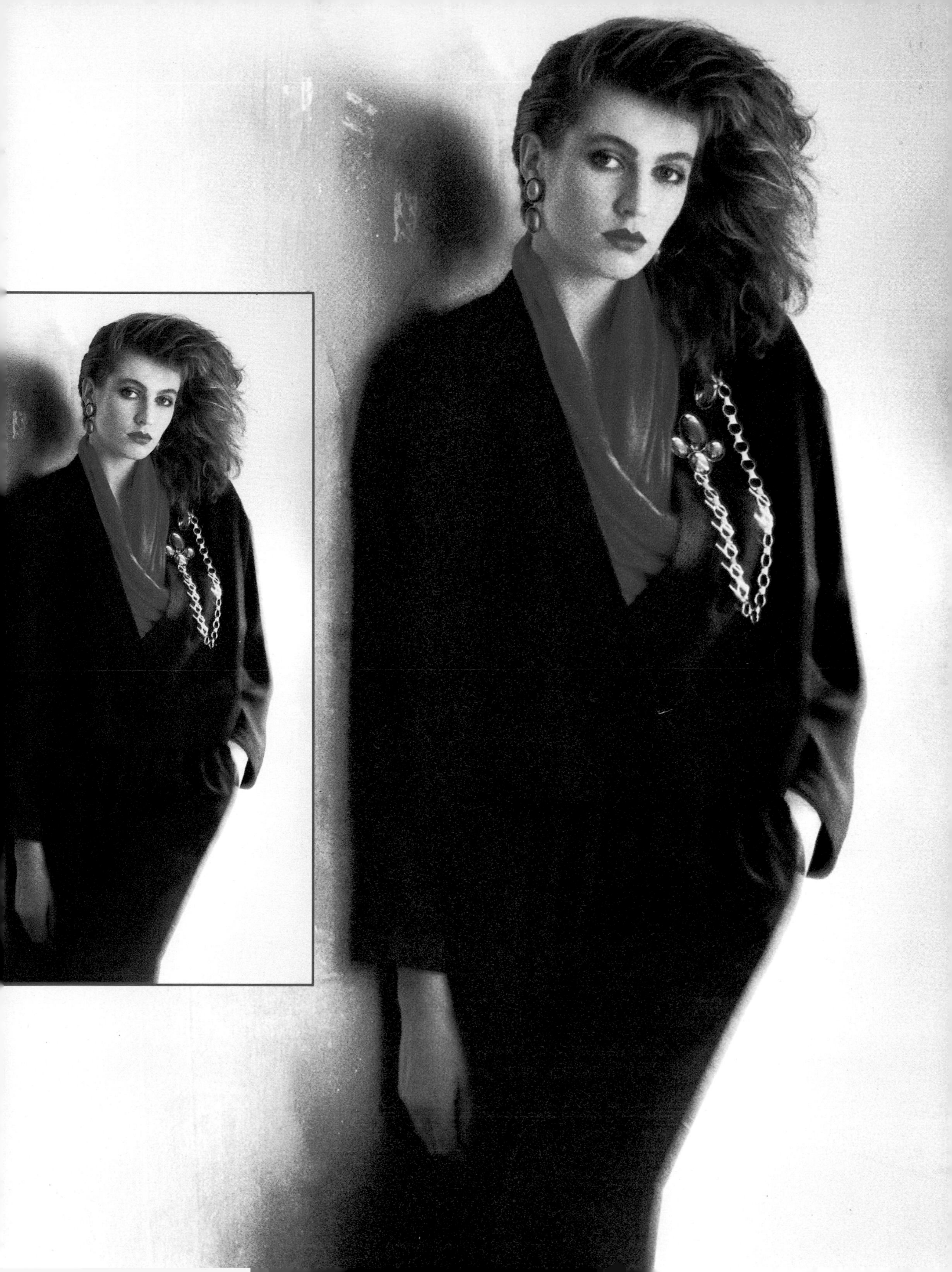

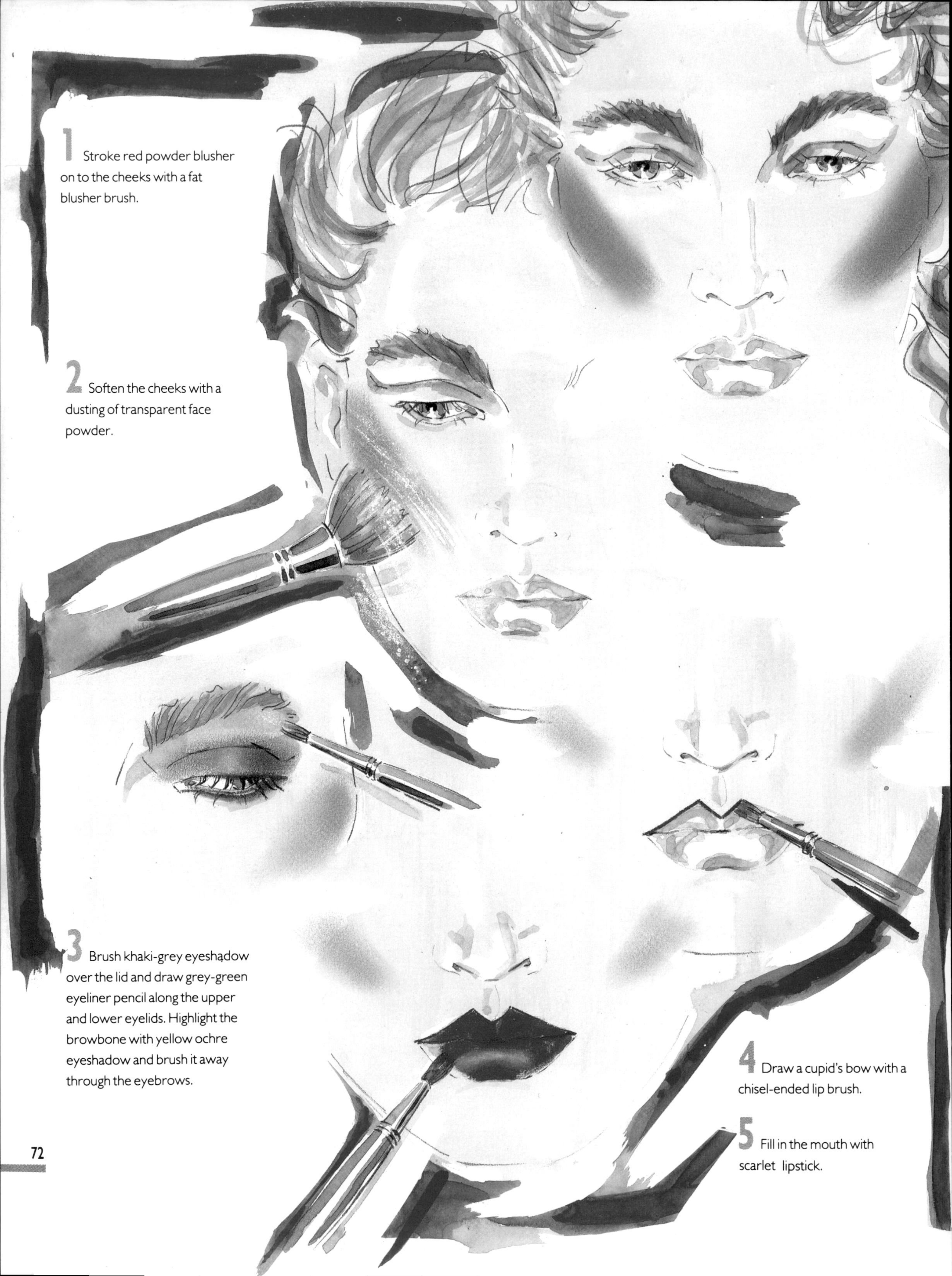

1 Stroke red powder blusher on to the cheeks with a fat blusher brush.

2 Soften the cheeks with a dusting of transparent face powder.

3 Brush khaki-grey eyeshadow over the lid and draw grey-green eyeliner pencil along the upper and lower eyelids. Highlight the browbone with yellow ochre eyeshadow and brush it away through the eyebrows.

4 Draw a cupid's bow with a chisel-ended lip brush.

5 Fill in the mouth with scarlet lipstick.

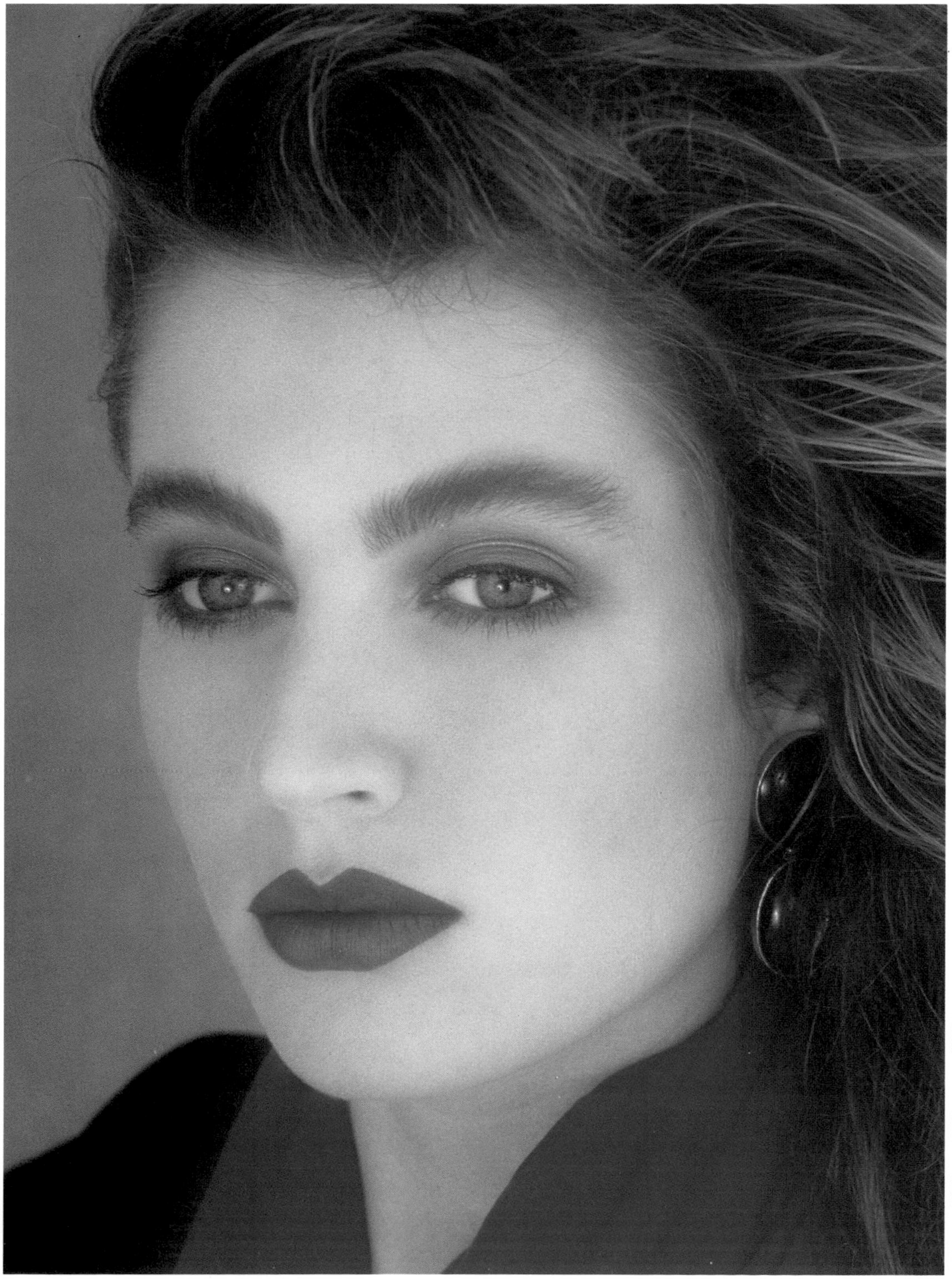

This sexy evening look started with a pale foundation and face powder. Red powder blusher was stroked on to the cheeks with a fat blusher brush. The effect of the blush was softened by a generous dusting of transparent face powder. Khaki-grey eyeshadow was brushed over the lid, and a grey-green eyeliner pencil was drawn along the upper and lower eyelids to give the eyes a slightly downward droop. The same grey mixed with the khaki deepens the shadow at the outer corner of the eye. I used yellow ochre eyeshadow to highlight the area below the eyebrow, and blended a touch of it into the centre of the upper lid. A line of dark grey kohl pencil was drawn on the inner rim of the lower lid. The eyes were finished with black mascara. A sharp cupid's bow was drawn with a chisel-ended lip brush, and the mouth filled in with scarlet lipstick.

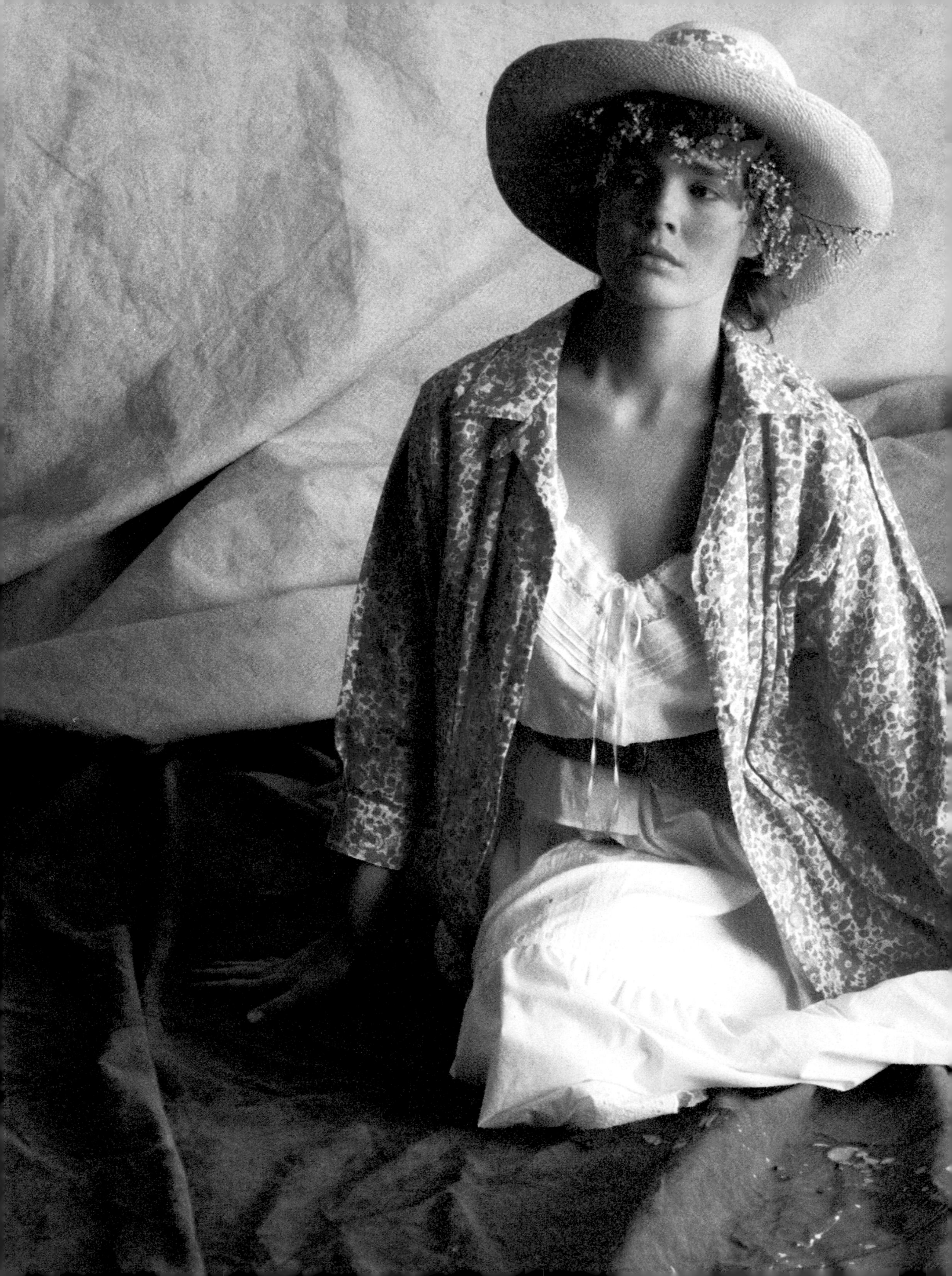

BLUES COUNTRY

Blue looks cool on the hottest summer's day. Floral sprigs around a pale and pretty face have a nostalgic air; the look is simple and casual — just the thing for a picnic in a meadow. The plain and country-fresh straw hat carries the only adornments, a swathe of matching fabric and sprays of flowers.

This fresh, young look is very flattering to the creamy pale skin of a redhead, and is inspired by the blue of our model, Wendy's, eyes. The temptation is to go for a totally blue eye make-up too — but then the eyes lose out. The palest of pastel lilacs enhances the delicate tones of the face without being obtrusive.

'For this look, very little needed to be done to the hair. I drew it back into a ponytail and coaxed the ends to work loose in a wispy fashion around Wendy's face. We clipped sprays of silk flowers into the hair and put the hat on top.' **J F**

Top, Skirt and Hat: Ralph Lauren · Coat-dress: Margaret Howell

The fresh, country face is achieved with a natural tone base, very lightly powdered. I applied a pale lavender eyeshadow all over the eyelid — at its darkest next to the lashes and blended away to nothing at the eyebrow. A line of silvery turquoise eye pencil was drawn through the lower lashes and softened with a brush below the eye. A touch of iridescent bluish-white highlighter is brushed on the centre of the eyelid and on the browbone to add sheen. Royal blue mascara on the lashes flatters the eye colour, and a touch of mascara on a thin eyeliner brush is used to draw a fine line very close to the top lashes. Pinky powder blusher on the centre of the cheeks gives a young look. I used sugar pink lipstick without a defining line to make a pale, soft mouth.

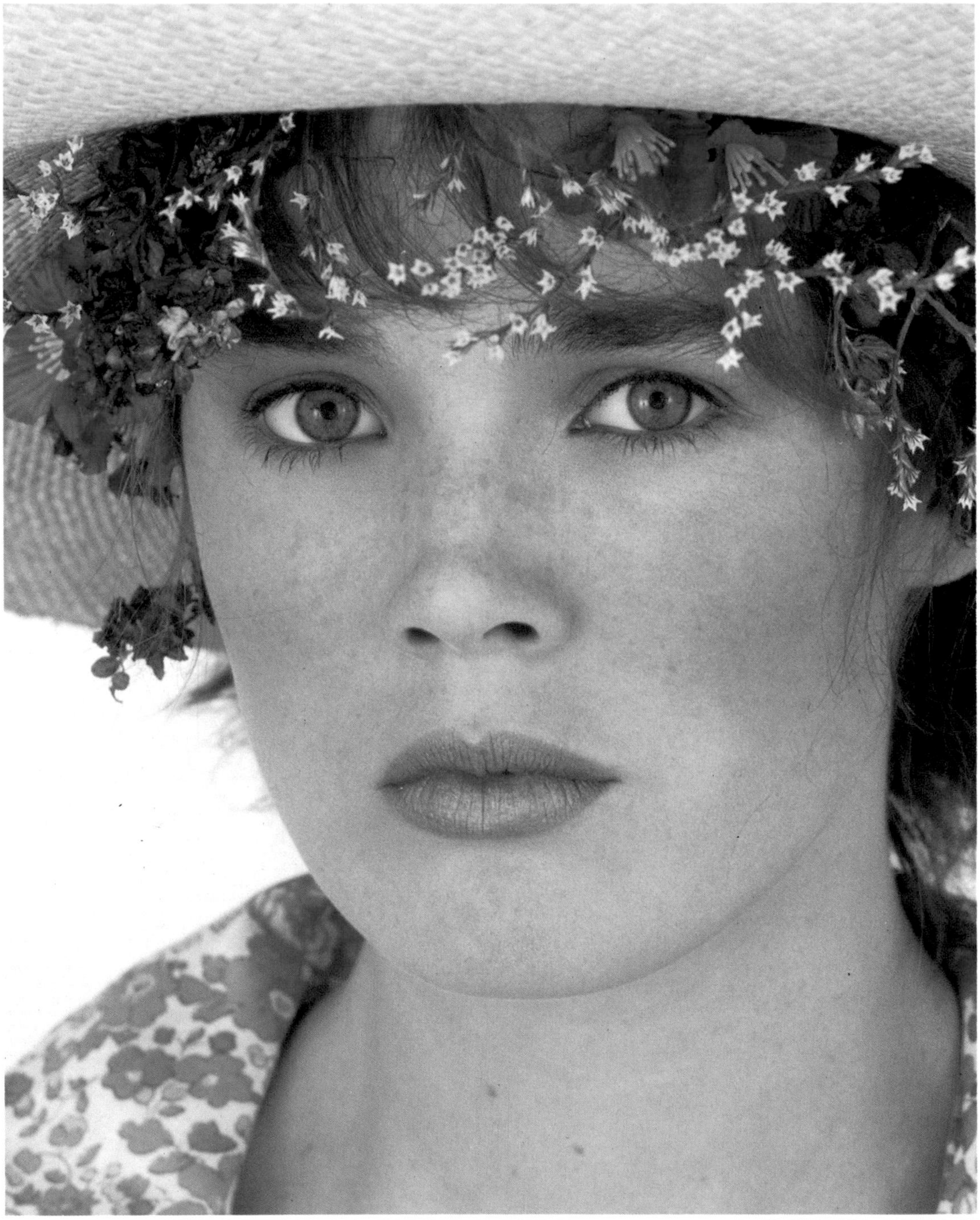

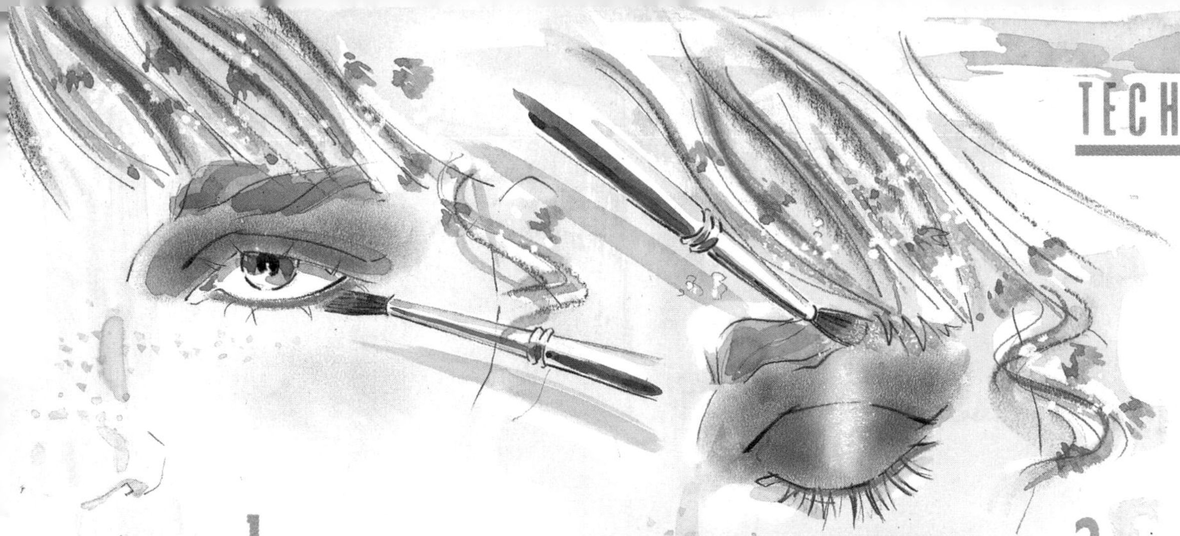

1 Apply pale lavender eyeshadow all over the eyelid, blending away to the brow. Draw a line of silvery turquoise eye pencil through the lower lashes, softening it with a brush.

2 Brush iridescent highlighter through the centre of the eyelid and on the browbone.

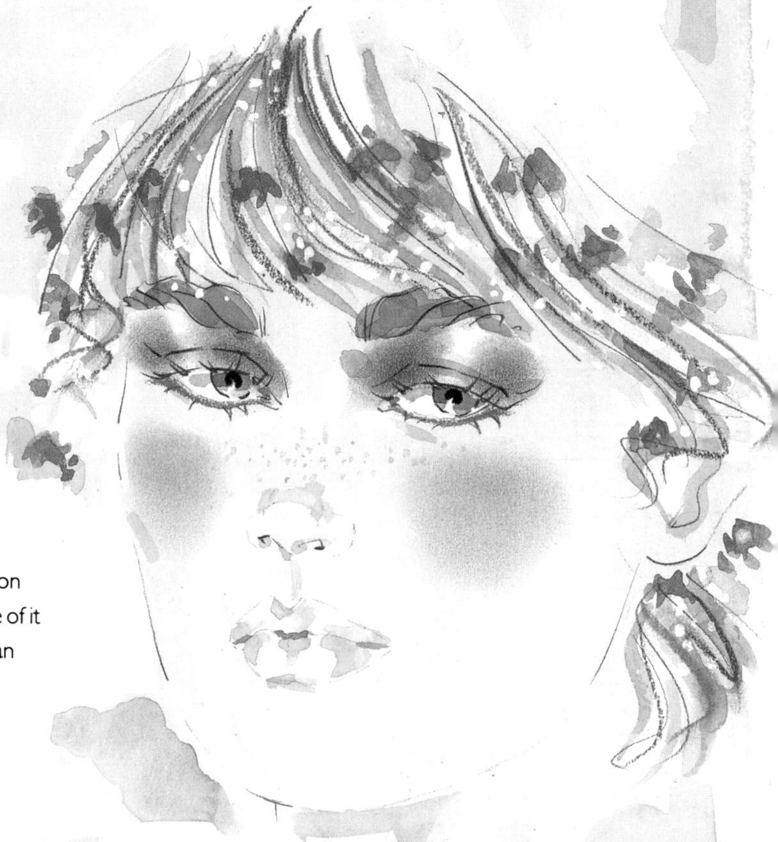

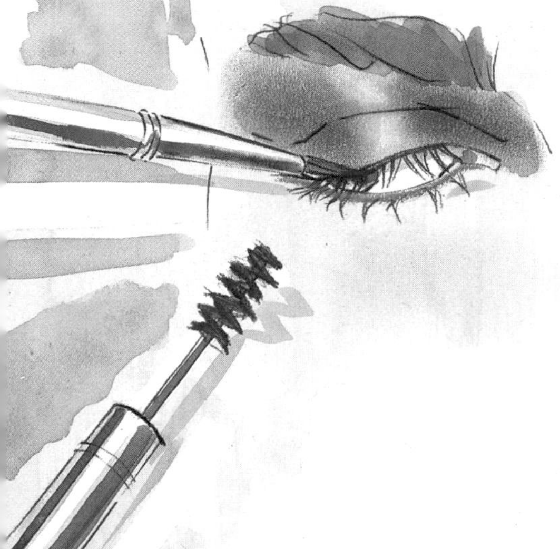

3 Use royal blue mascara on the lashes, drawing a fine line of it through the top lashes with an eyeliner brush.

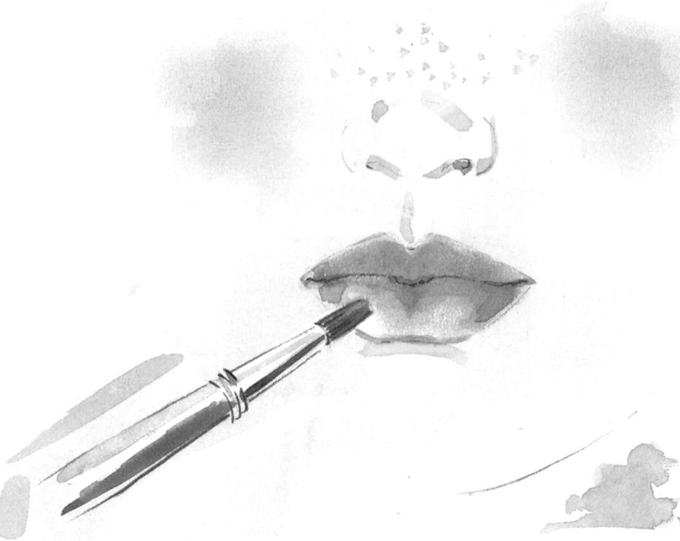

4 Fluff pinky powder blusher on the centre of the cheeks.

5 Apply sugar pink lipstick without an outline.

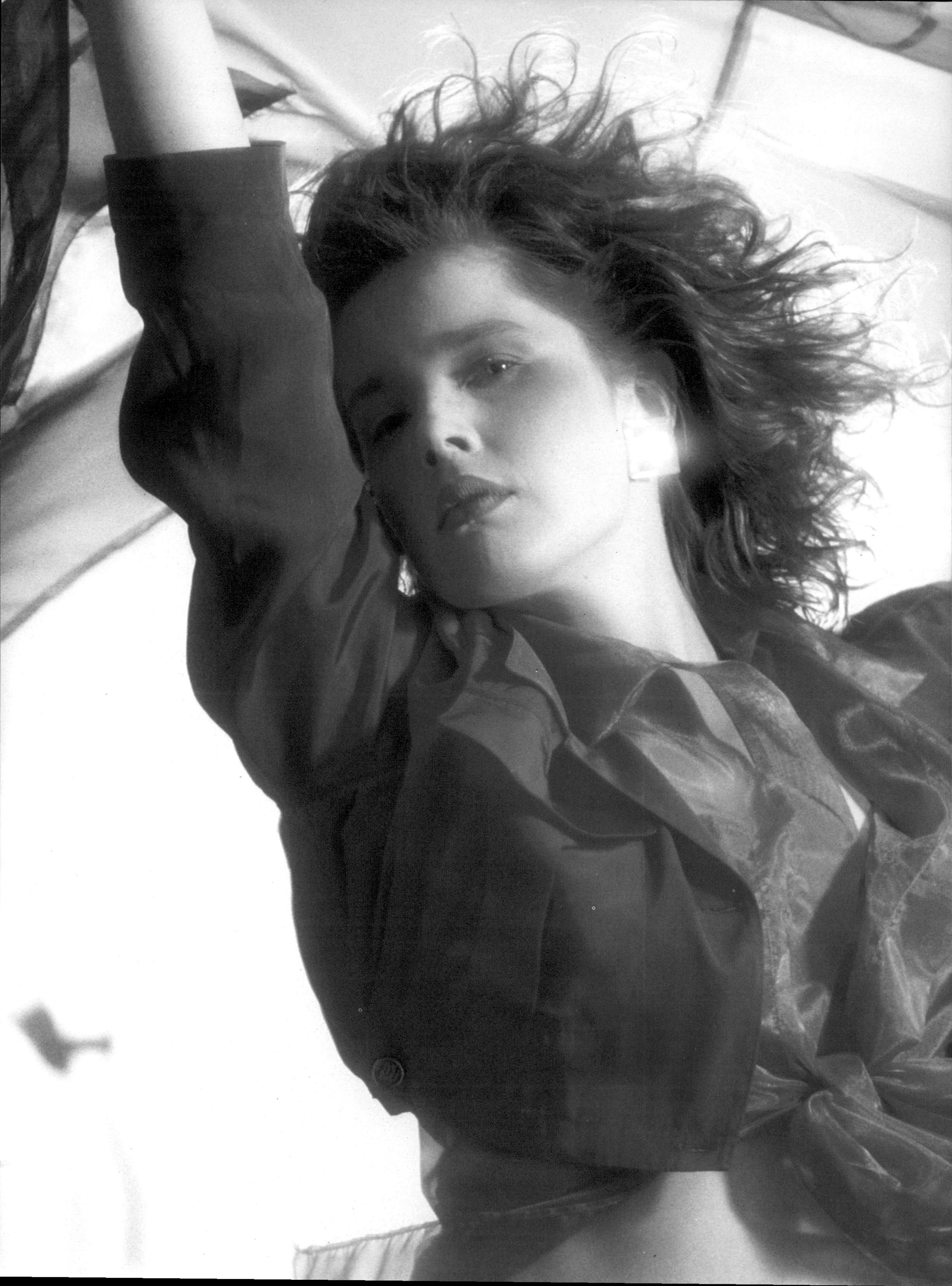

Pink Suit: Gaultier at Browns · Orange shirt & bra-top: Whistles · Earrings: Detail

Orange is sizzling. Teamed with hot pink it is completely over-the-top and fun. Wear this evening extravaganza if you want to be noticed: filmy, silky fabrics — which happen to be easy-to-wear — in sensational shades.

Orange and pink, you will have been told, clash with your hair as well as with each other, but that's what you want: dynamic interaction of colour from head to foot.

Make-up has to be something really inspired if the clothes are not to take over. A zappy harlequin effect breaks every known rule, creating a piece of art on the pale canvas of your face. One rule only remains: however bright the colours, the application must still be ultra-careful. This make-up takes time because blending is a slow business — but the reward is a final effect with the quality of a painting.

'First I set Wendy's hair on large rollers using plenty of setting lotion. When it was dry and wound off the rollers, I worked wax on my hands and through the hair, then brushed it, working upwards, into a wild-looking mane. Finally lightning flashes of red fluorescent hair gel were streaked at the front.' **J F**

FUCHSIA SHOCK

1 Using a big brush, apply orange powder eyeshadow all over one eyelid, winging it out at the side and up towards the temple. Repeat with pink shadow on the other eye. Apply the opposite colour in each case to form a curved triangle of blush below the eye.

2 Outline the lower lid of each eye with pencil in a colour to match the cheek.

3 Mix powder eyeshadow with white powder and brush it into the brows to soften them.

4 Outline the lips with orange and pink pencils to form a chequerboard pattern, then fill in with the appropriate colour lipstick.

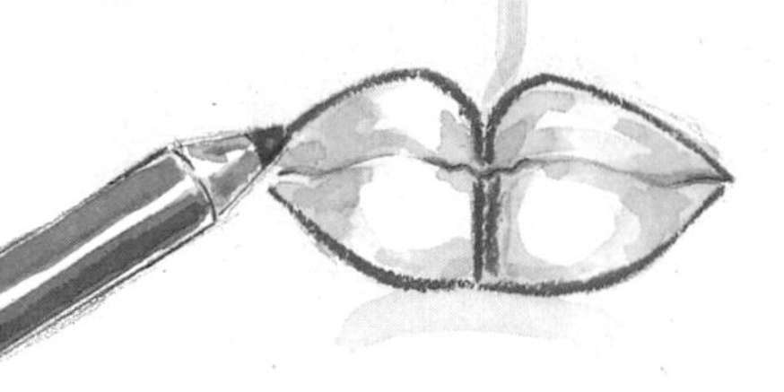

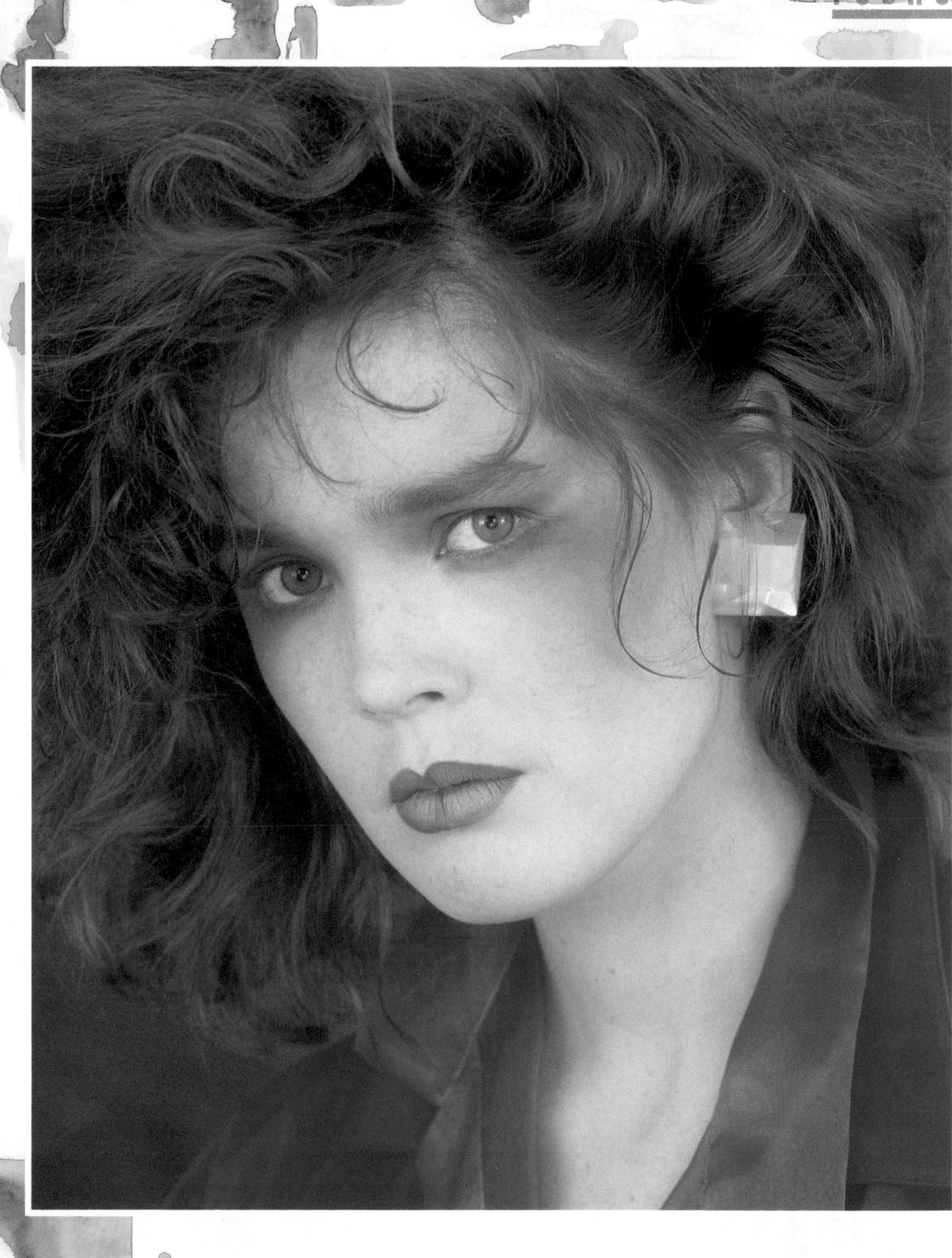

The harlequin face is extremely pale – skin-toned foundation lightened by mixing a white base into it. I used white alone over the eye area. The base is 'set' with pale loose face powder. Orange powder eyeshadow is brushed all over one eyelid, winging out at the side and up towards the temple. The same thing is repeated with bright strong pink on the other eye.

The pink and orange are blended to fade into each other over the bridge of the nose. The opposite colour in each case was used below the eyes, tapering down the cheeks to form a triangular blush shape. I outlined the eyes in pencil matching the shade used on the cheek – pink on pink, orange on orange. Mascara was applied on the same principle. I brushed eye shadow blended with white powder into the eyebrows. Outline the lips with orange and pink lip pencils in chequerboard pattern. Fill in with two different lipsticks.

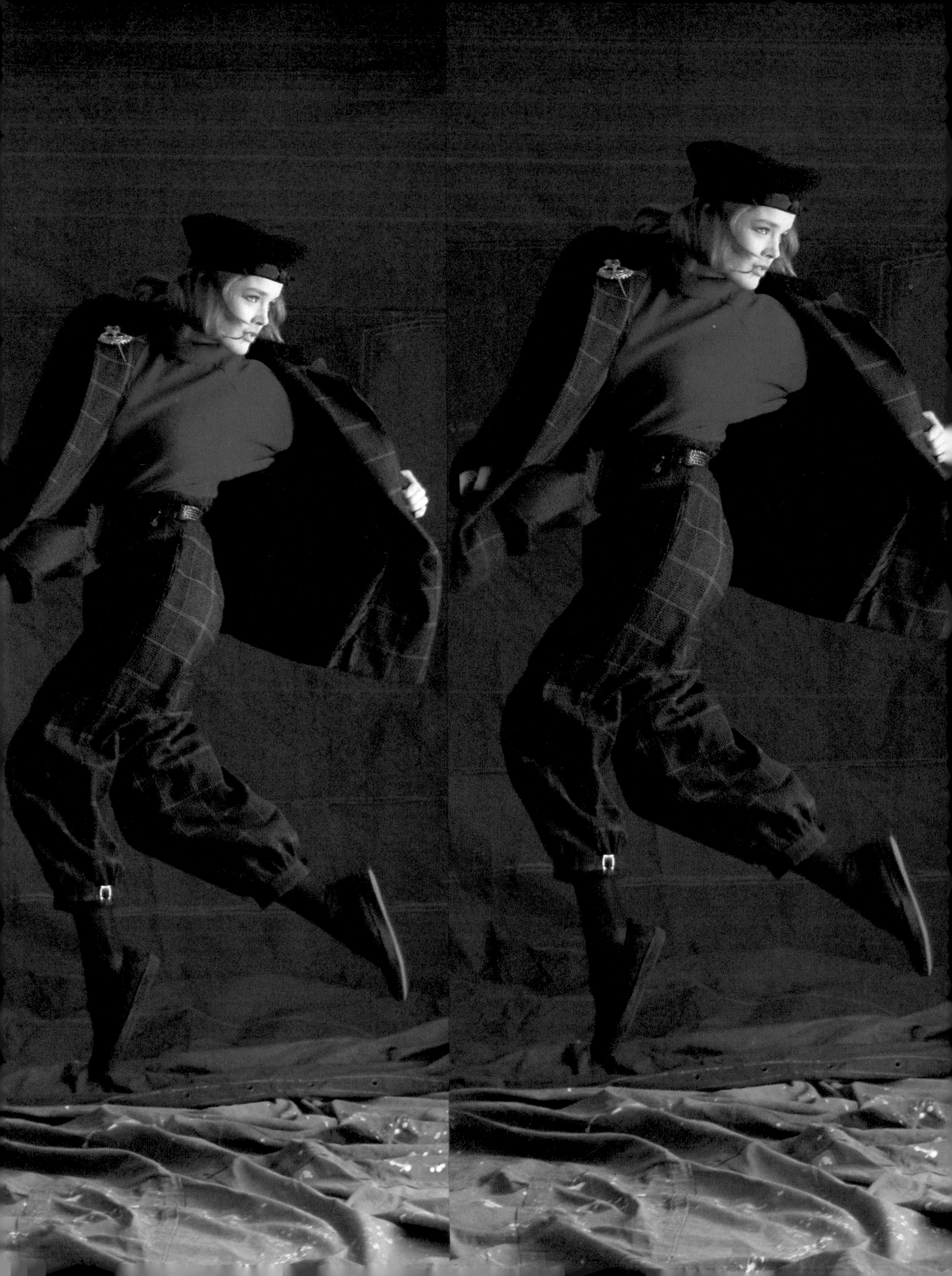

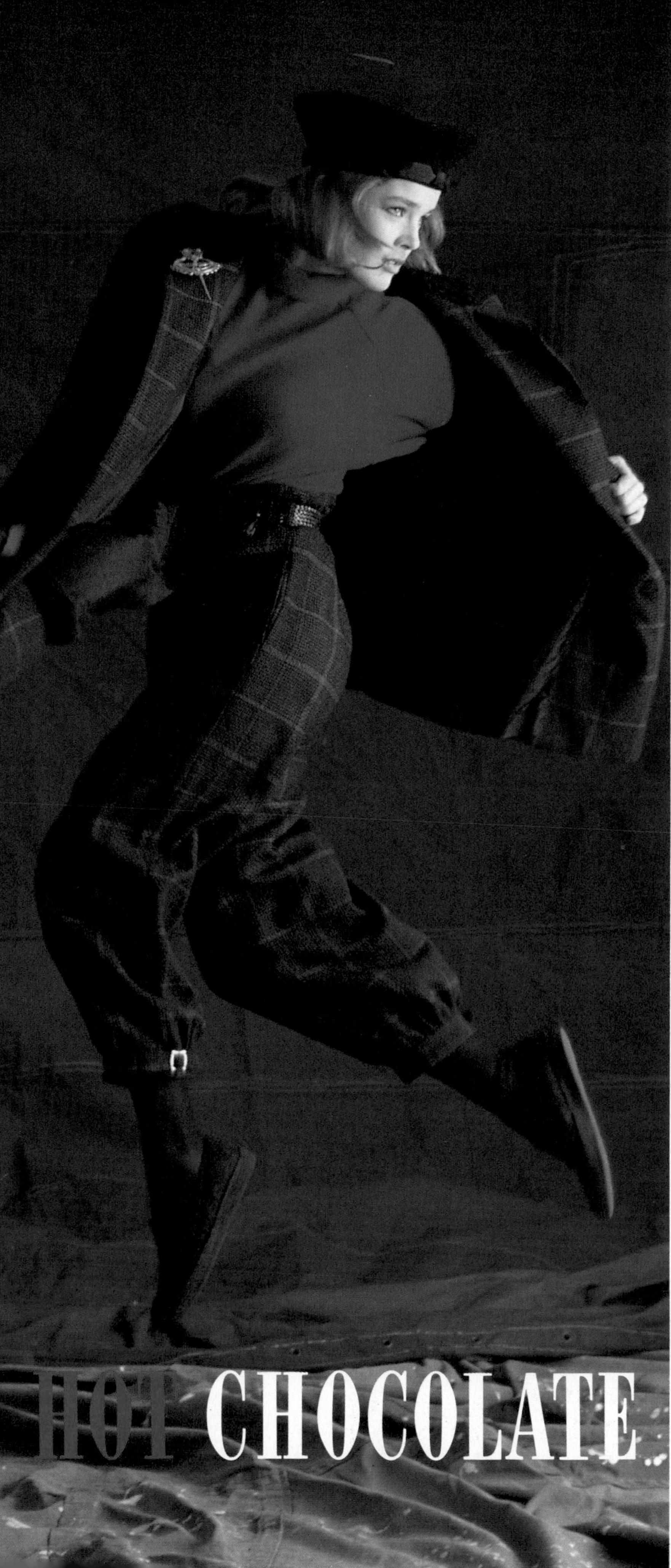

HOT CHOCOLATE

Clothes: Betty Jackson · Hat: Viv Knowland · Brooch: Monty Don ·

Brown is a good choice for the working girl. A simple well-cut suit such as this is a modern classic that can be worn anywhere, and by almost every figure type. What lifts it to the height of Parisian chic are the clever accessories: the emphatic hat, the clinching belt, the imposing brooch. What makes it both vivid and warm is the ruby red of the jumper, picking up the red check pattern of the suit.

The make-up is a working girl's dream, quick to apply and easy to remember. The theme of brown on eyes, cheeks and lips shows how you can wear this colour without looking dull, secure in the knowledge that you look self-assured and *soignée* but not over made-up.

'The aim here was to make the hair look as smooth as a sheet of glass. Setting lotion was combed through first and then the hair was carefully blowdried. I worked in sections, holding the hair taut with a round brush. Lastly I put large heated curlers in the ends for a moment to get a smooth finish.' **J F**

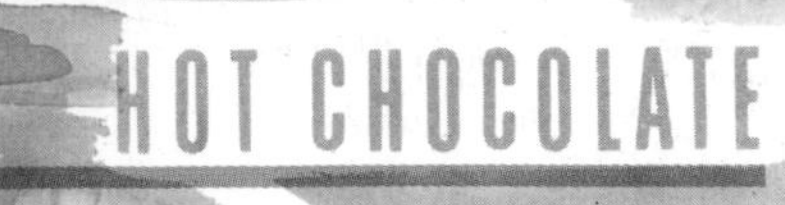

HOT CHOCOLATE

Start with a pale, creamy base and set with powder. For a redhead any colour of brown eyeshadow will do (except one with a grey tone), brushed over the entire eye area. The colour is more concentrated at the outer corner of the eye and winging outwards. With a brush, blend the shadow away to nothing up to the eyebrow. Under the lower eyelid the same shadow is smoothed, with a brush, to a smoky line. Cream coloured highlight is blended on the browbone, and the eyes are defined with a thin line of black. The lightest touch of brown blusher is dusted on the cheekbones. Use a brown pencil to outline the lips very lightly and fill in with light brown lipstick, using a brush.

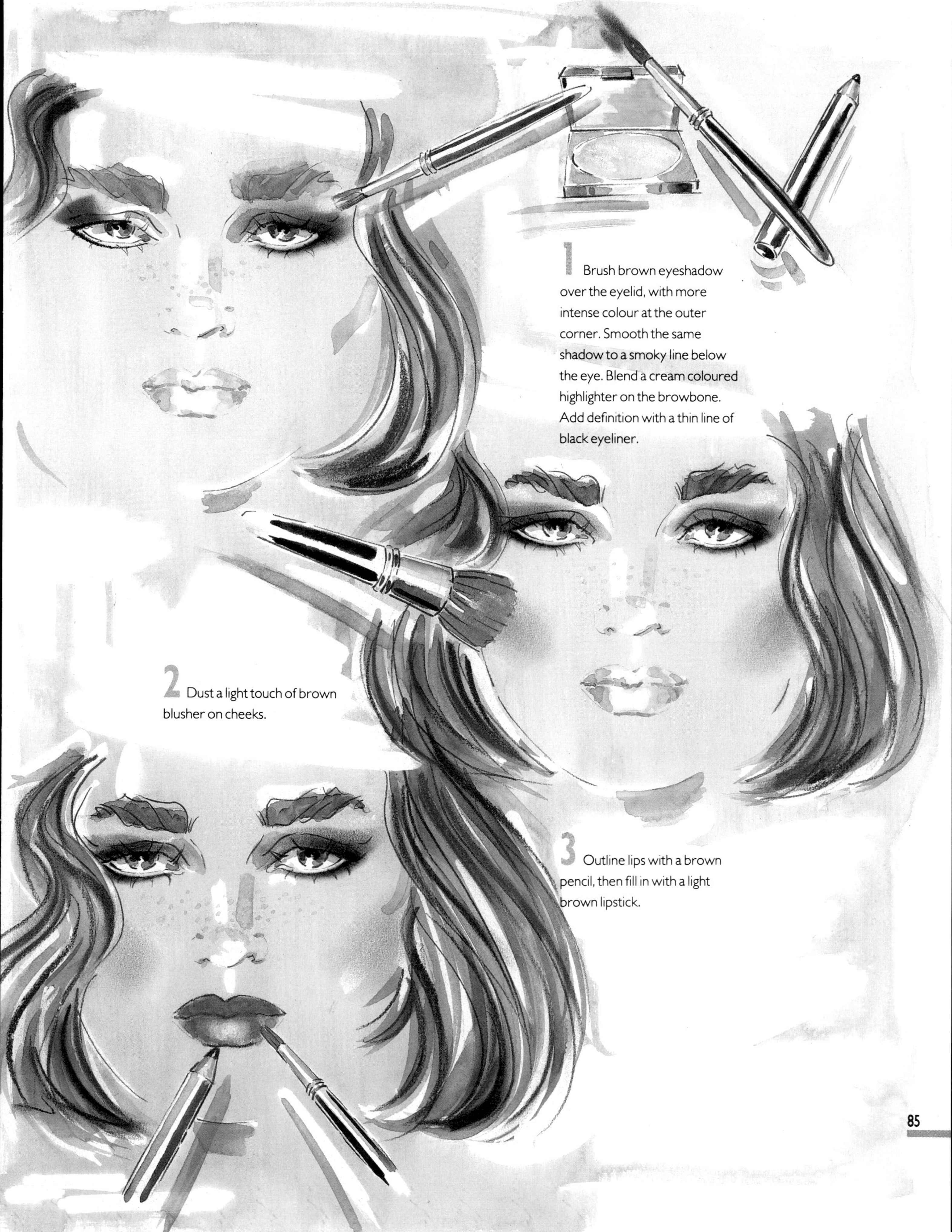

1 Brush brown eyeshadow over the eyelid, with more intense colour at the outer corner. Smooth the same shadow to a smoky line below the eye. Blend a cream coloured highlighter on the browbone. Add definition with a thin line of black eyeliner.

2 Dust a light touch of brown blusher on cheeks.

3 Outline lips with a brown pencil, then fill in with a light brown lipstick.

CREAM CRACKERS

Cream is fresh – and sporty. Against pale skin, unless carefully handled, it can contribute to a washed-out look. You can take it, because the contrast with your strong colouring can be sensational. This simple, cable-stitch sweater striped with navy, teamed with white shirt, skirt, socks and shoes – a strip of Jane's bare brown leg showing between sock and hemline – actually looks very elegant.

Make-up against cream needs to be emphatic but uncomplicated: sultry smoky eyes and a red lipstick give a daytime look both subtle and bold, which manages to mix sport with glamour.

'The sleek schoolboy hairstyle is achieved by thoroughly dampening the hair and combing it through, using hair wax or hair gel. It is smoothed and shaped with comb and hands. The front roll is loosely curled and shaped with the comb and fingers. Mousse is stroked on to the back of the hair. Tie a chiffon scarf tightly round while it is still damp so that it doesn't lift up as it dries.' **J F**

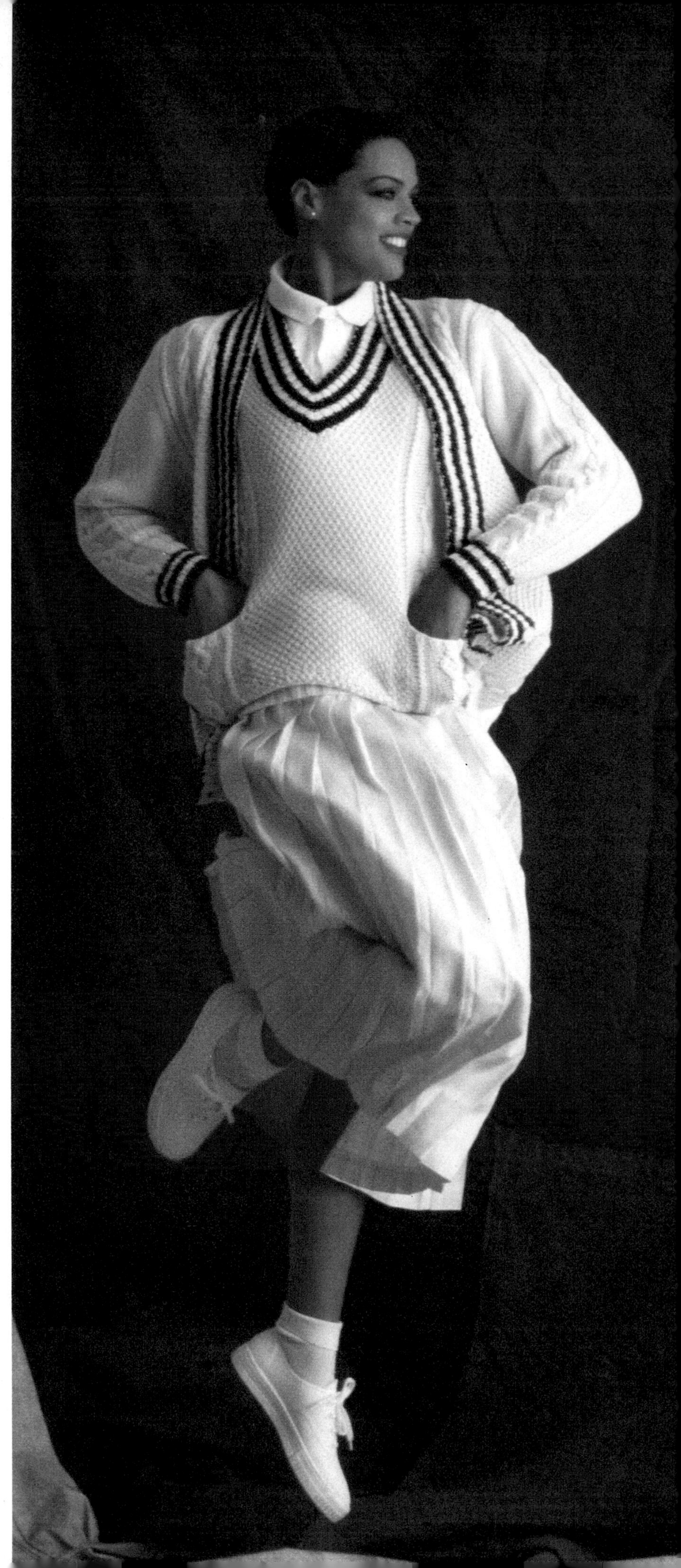

Clothes: Ralph Lauren · Plimsolls: Whistles

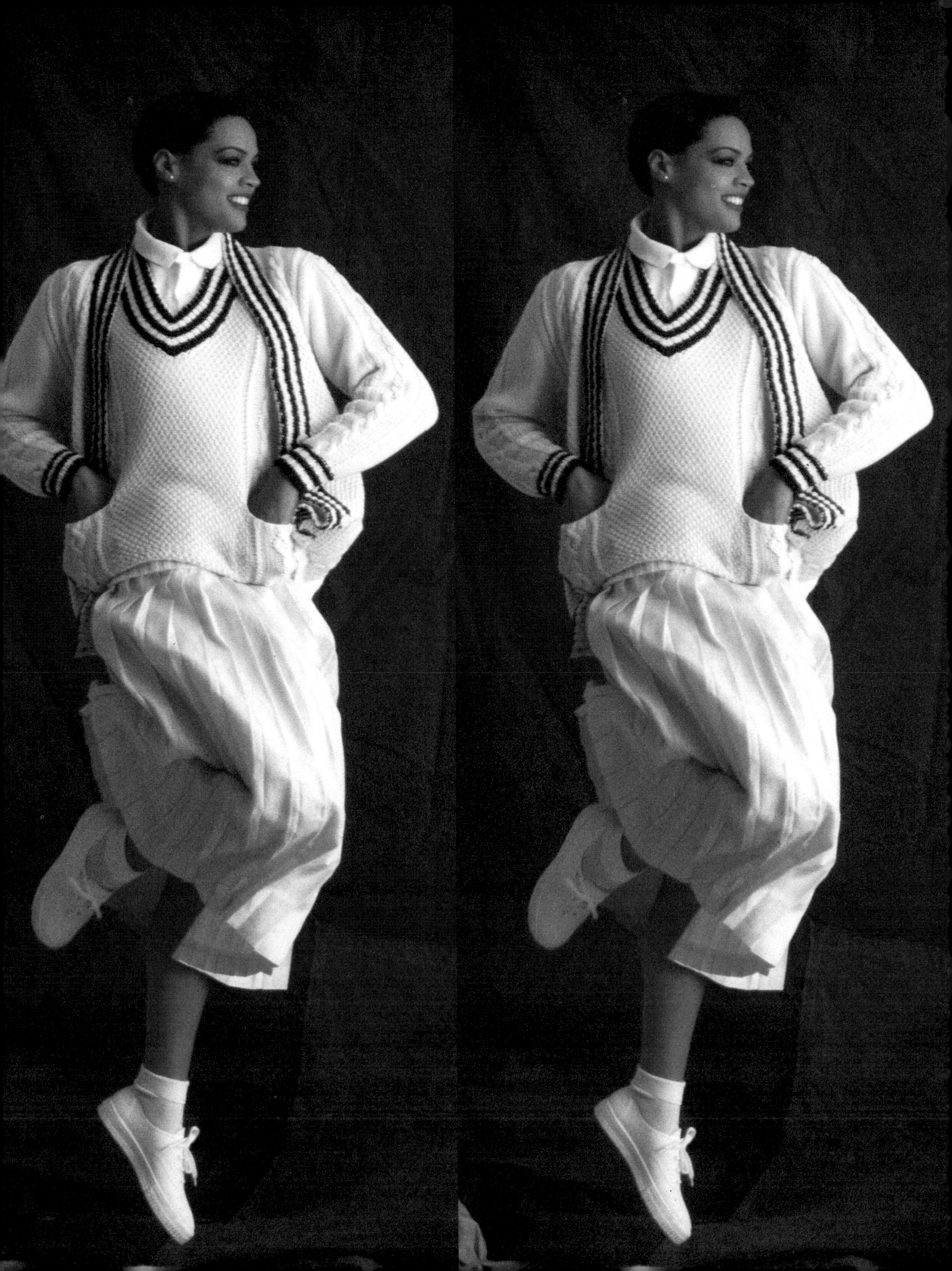

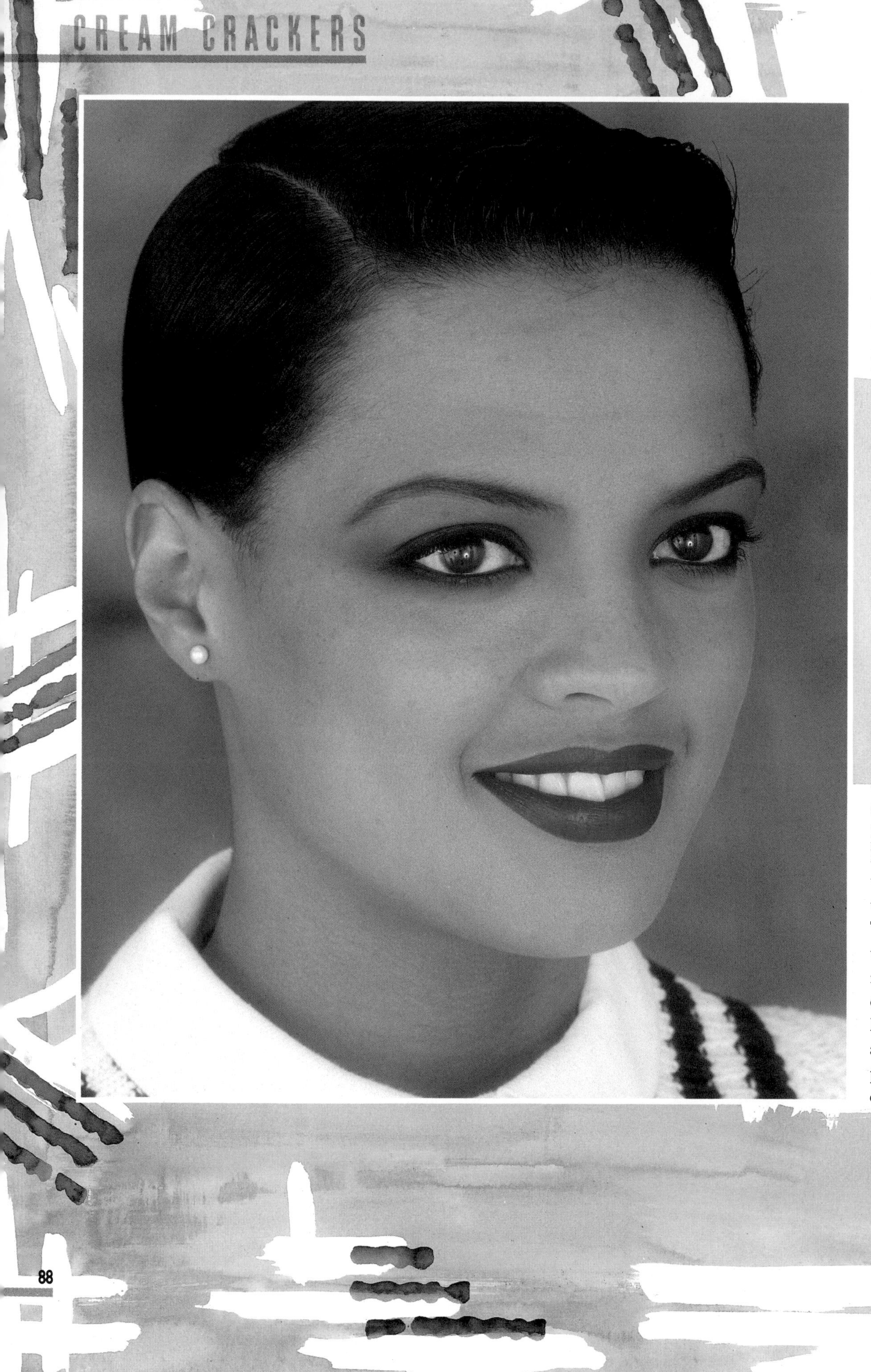

An exact match of skin tone is achieved by mixing two or more foundations together on the back of your hand. A basic skin colour mixed with a pinker or more yellow tone will give you the result you want. I drew a fat, dark brown pencil line along the upper eyelid and blended it with a brush, setting it with a light dusting of face powder. Brown powder eyeshadow was brushed towards the outer corner of the eyebrow, blended very lightly down the bridge of the nose to slim it, and under the eye for a smudgy effect. I used black cake eyeshadow on a brush to emphasize the outer corners of the upper lid and as an eyeliner. Brown kohl pencil was drawn along the inner rim of the lower lid. Pink highlight was used on the browbone. The eyebrows were shaped and filled in with a dark brown pencil. The eyes were finished with two coats of black mascara. I outlined and coloured the lips with red lipstick. Finally I stroked a light dusting of red powder blusher on to the cheeks.

TECHNICAL TIPS

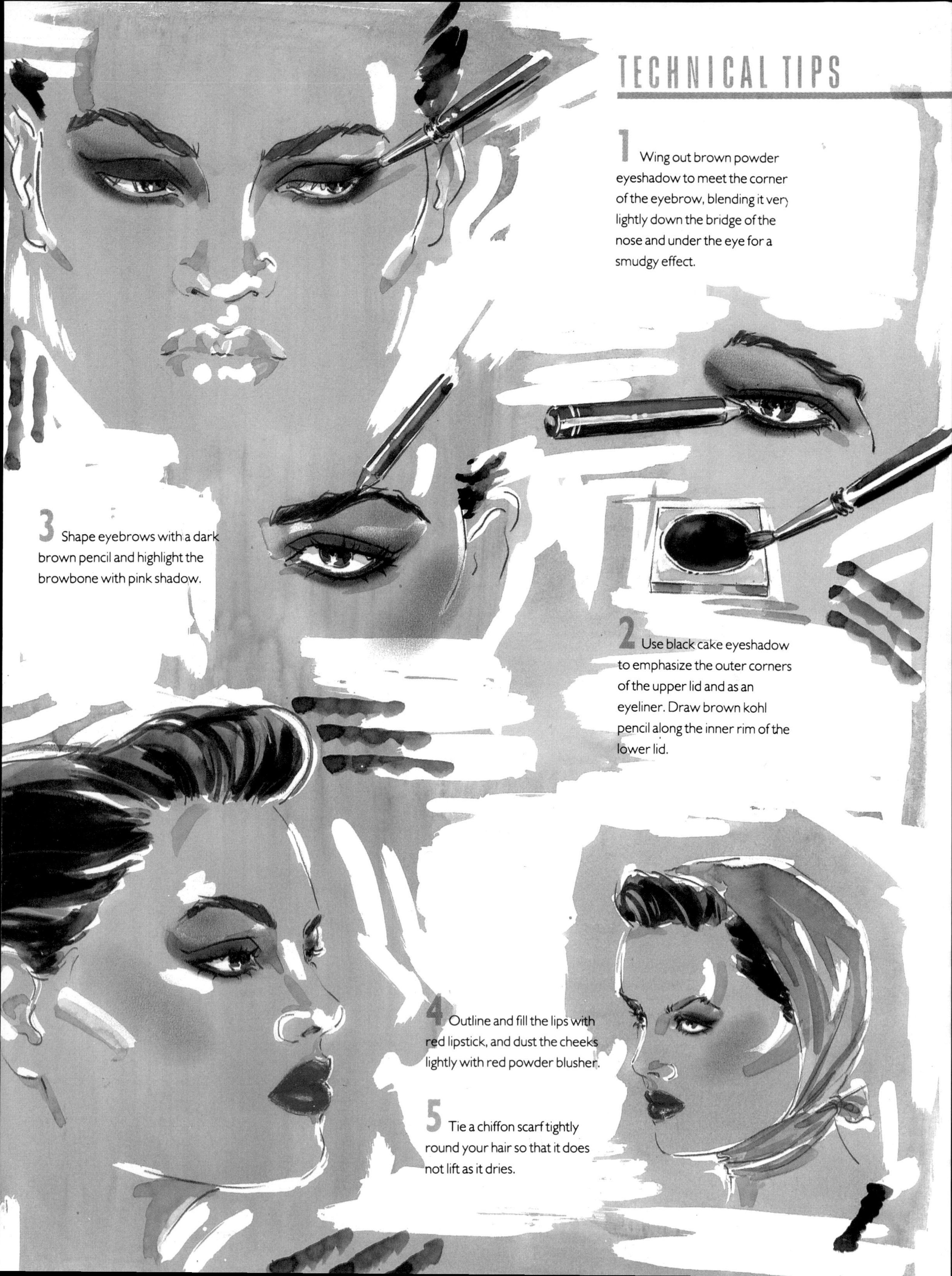

1 Wing out brown powder eyeshadow to meet the corner of the eyebrow, blending it very lightly down the bridge of the nose and under the eye for a smudgy effect.

2 Use black cake eyeshadow to emphasize the outer corners of the upper lid and as an eyeliner. Draw brown kohl pencil along the inner rim of the lower lid.

3 Shape eyebrows with a dark brown pencil and highlight the browbone with pink shadow.

4 Outline and fill the lips with red lipstick, and dust the cheeks lightly with red powder blusher.

5 Tie a chiffon scarf tightly round your hair so that it does not lift as it dries.

LIME LIGHT

Green offers an infinite variety of shades – some easy to wear, some not. Only you could get away with this daring mix of emerald and lime green and still look stunning. Whatever colour your skin is – from warm honey to deep mahogany – jewel-bright colours too strong for fairer skin glow against it and make you look terrific. The slinky sheath of a dress under a billowing diaphanous trench coat is a head-turning combination by anyone's standards, and you can carry it off with panache.

Your skin tone also means that you can wear intense colours on your face without looking gaudy. From purest white, which only suits dark skins, to the yellows and greens of this look, you have the entire range of the make-up palette to choose from.

'A glistening, sculptured look to hair is achieved by working in lots of hair wax or hair gel – or whatever product suits your hair. Pick up small strands, and then twist them with your fingers until you get the effect you want.' **J F**

Dress: Whistles · Coat: Gaultier at Browns · Earrings: Monty Don ·

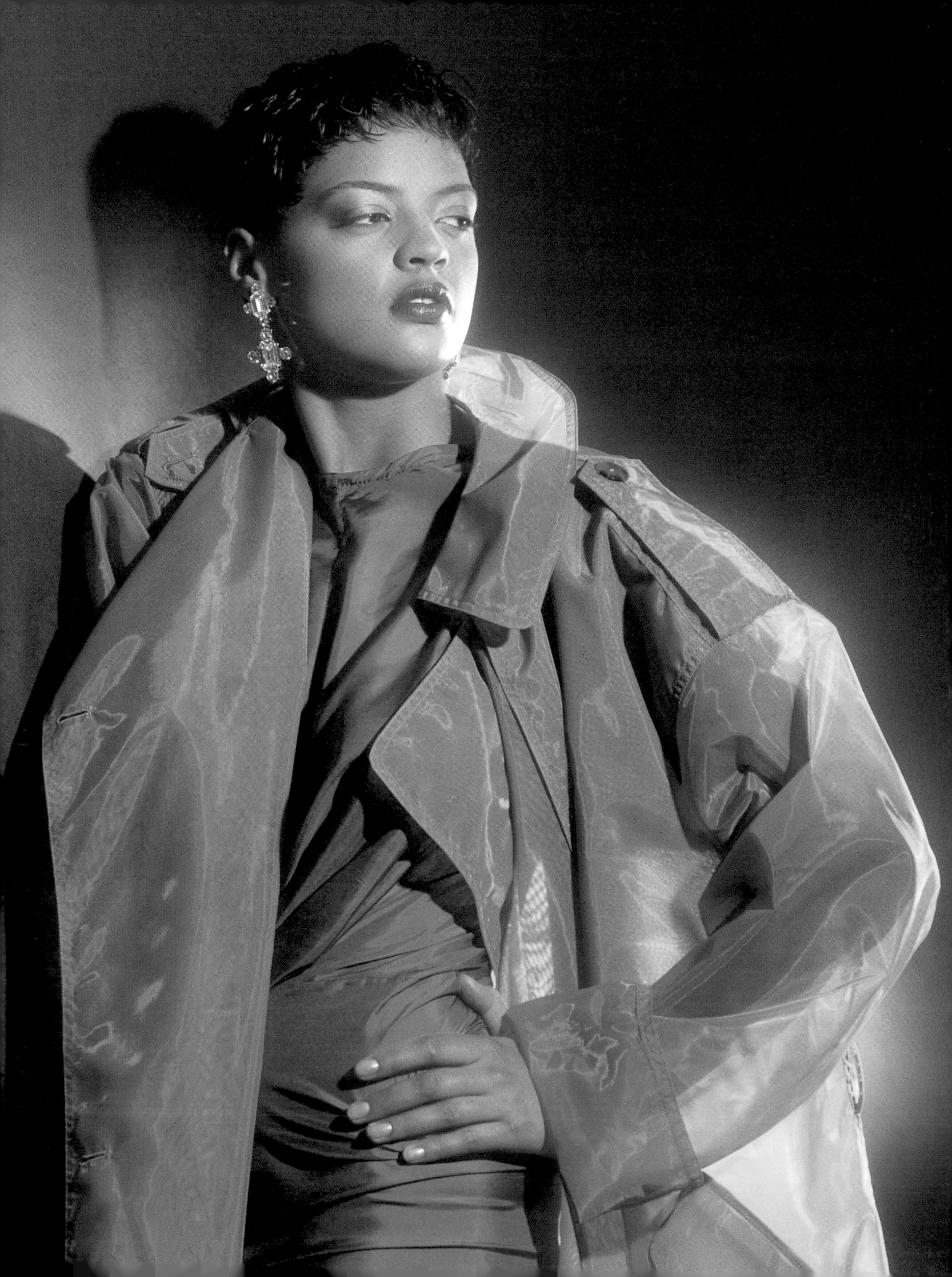

TECHNICAL TIPS

1 Apply dark green eyeshadow to the outer quarter of the eyelid and wing it upwards with a brush.

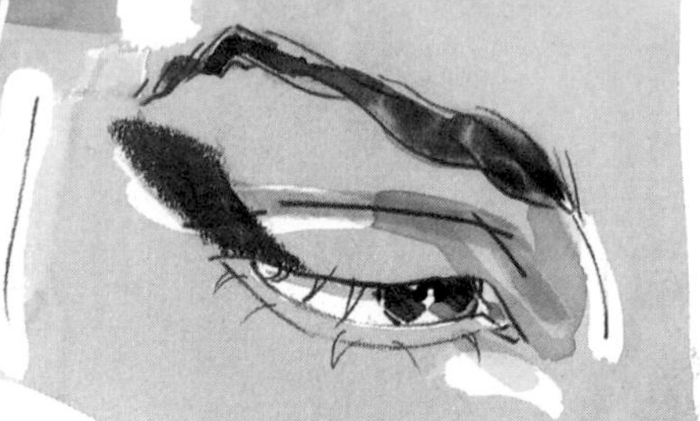

2 Cover the remaining three-quarters of the top lid with lime green powder eyeshadow and blend well.

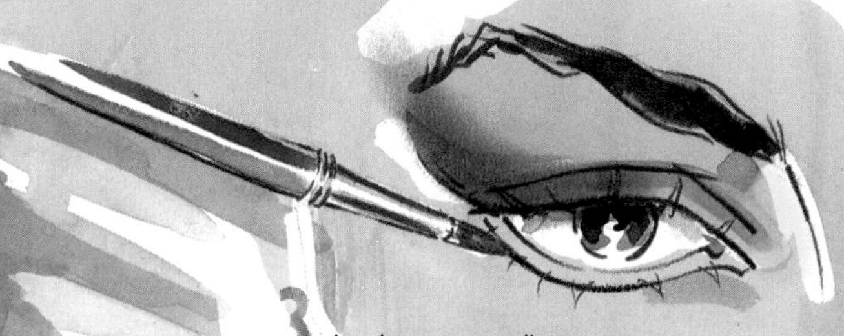

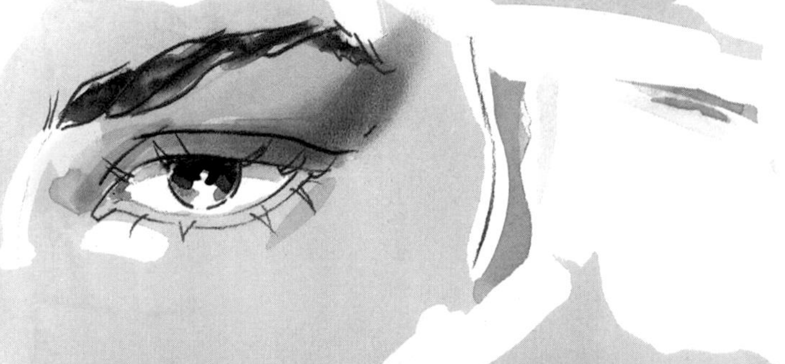

3 Apply green eyeliner top and bottom and wing it upwards.

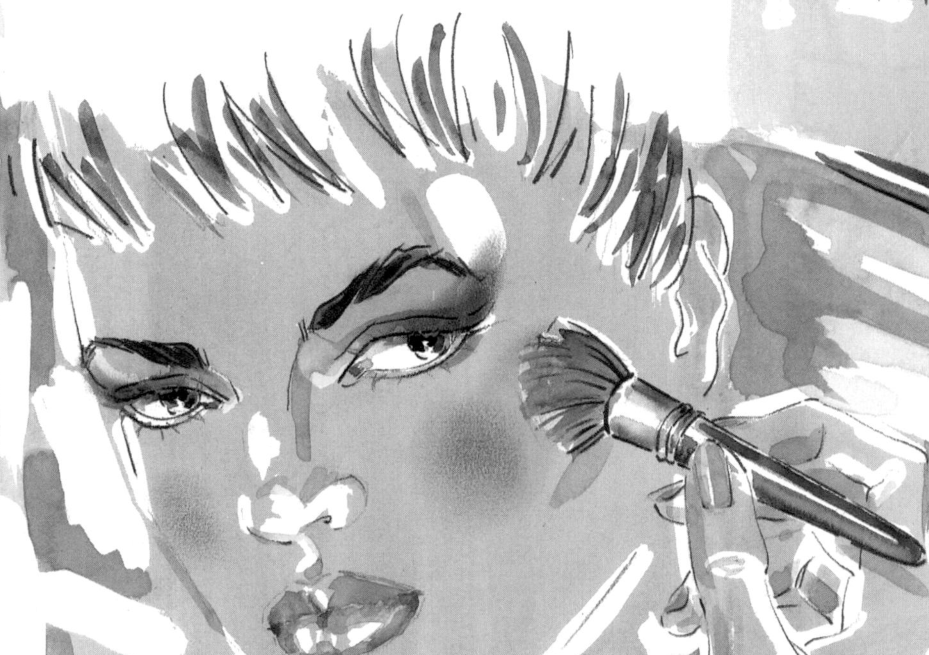

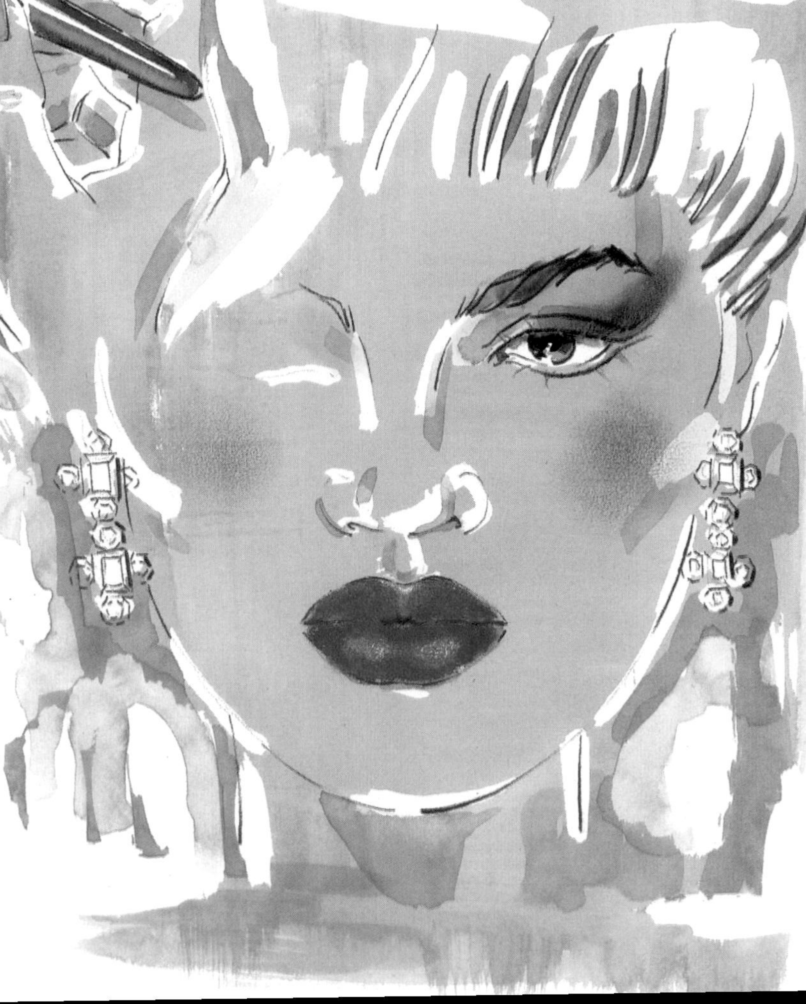

4 Fluff a pale green-yellow highlighter on to cheekbones with a blusher brush, with blue-pink blush on the cheeks.

5 Colour the mouth with raspberry pink lipstick.

I mixed a foundation base to the exact colour of Jane's skin using a 'suntan' tone foundation and a yellow toned one. The base was set with transparent powder. Dark green eyeshadow was drawn on the outer quarter of the eyelid and winged outwards with a brush. Lime green powder eyeshadow was applied three-quarters of the way along the top lid, and the join between the two was blended away. The colour was brushed upwards to the eyebrow and faded away towards the temple. A green eyeliner top and bottom was winged up at the sides to slant the eye, with dark green mascara to finish. A pale greeny-yellow highlighter was stroked high on the cheekbones with a blusher brush, with a blue-pink blush on the cheeks. The mouth was coloured with a raspberry pink lipstick.

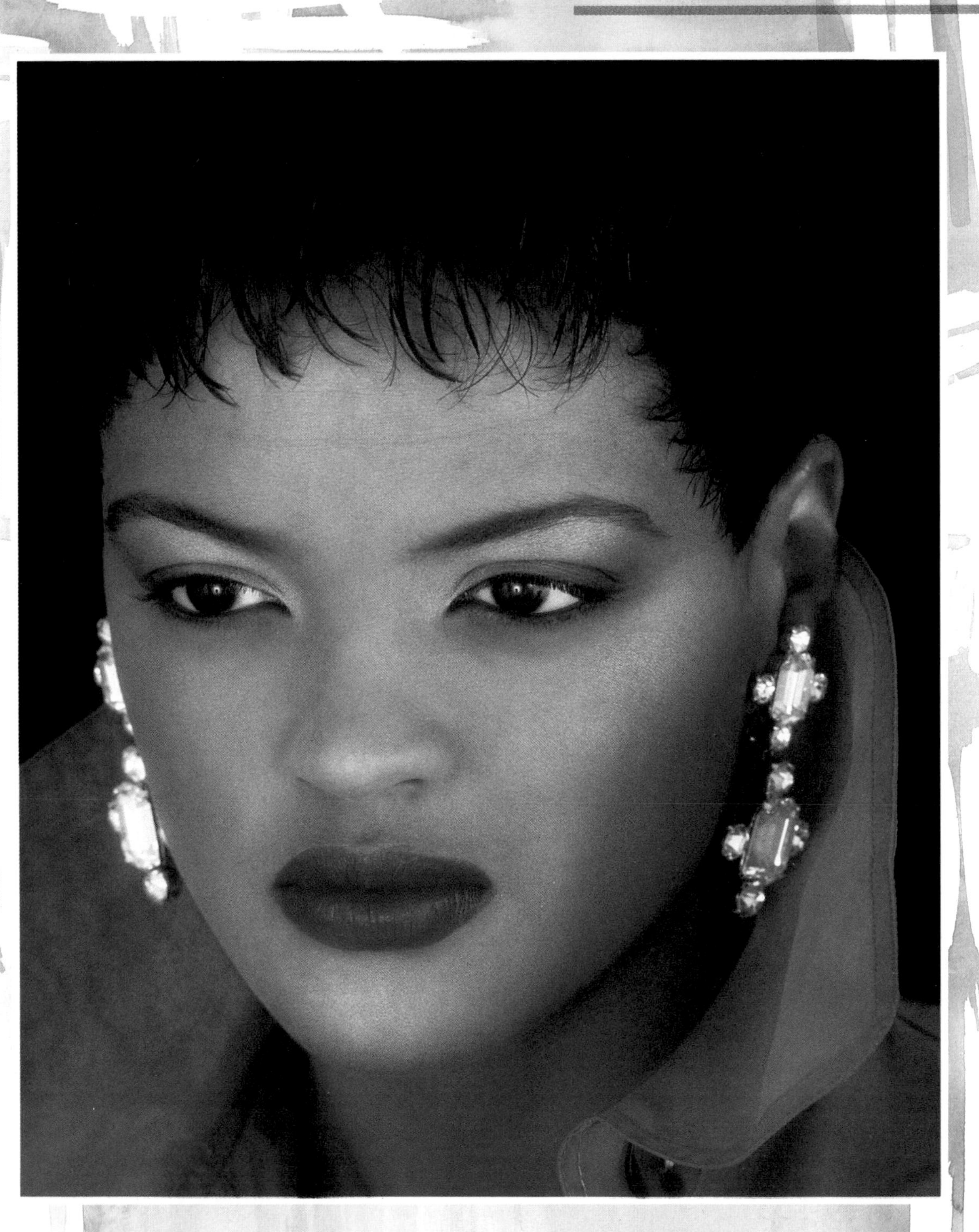

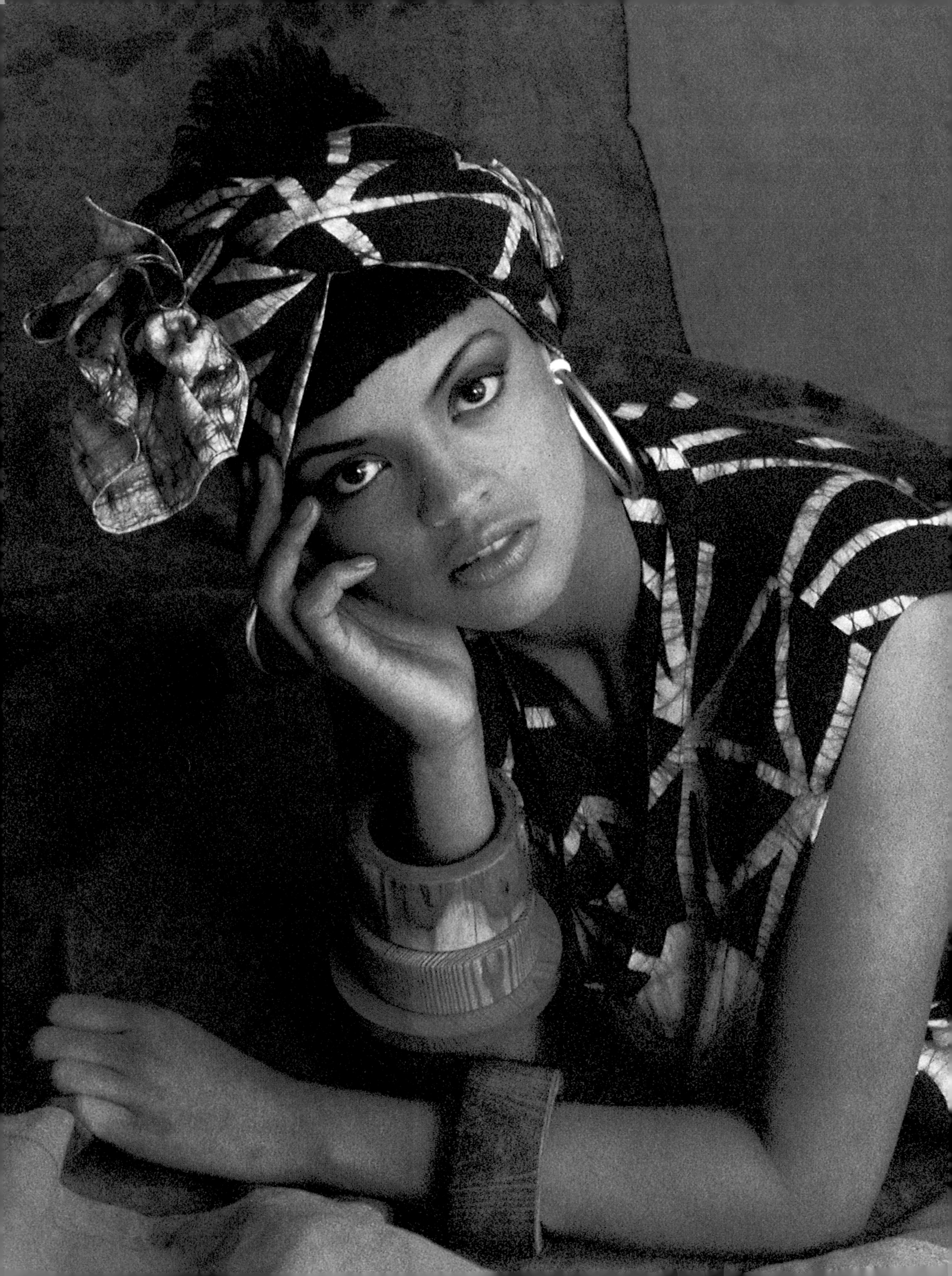

MOOD INDIGO

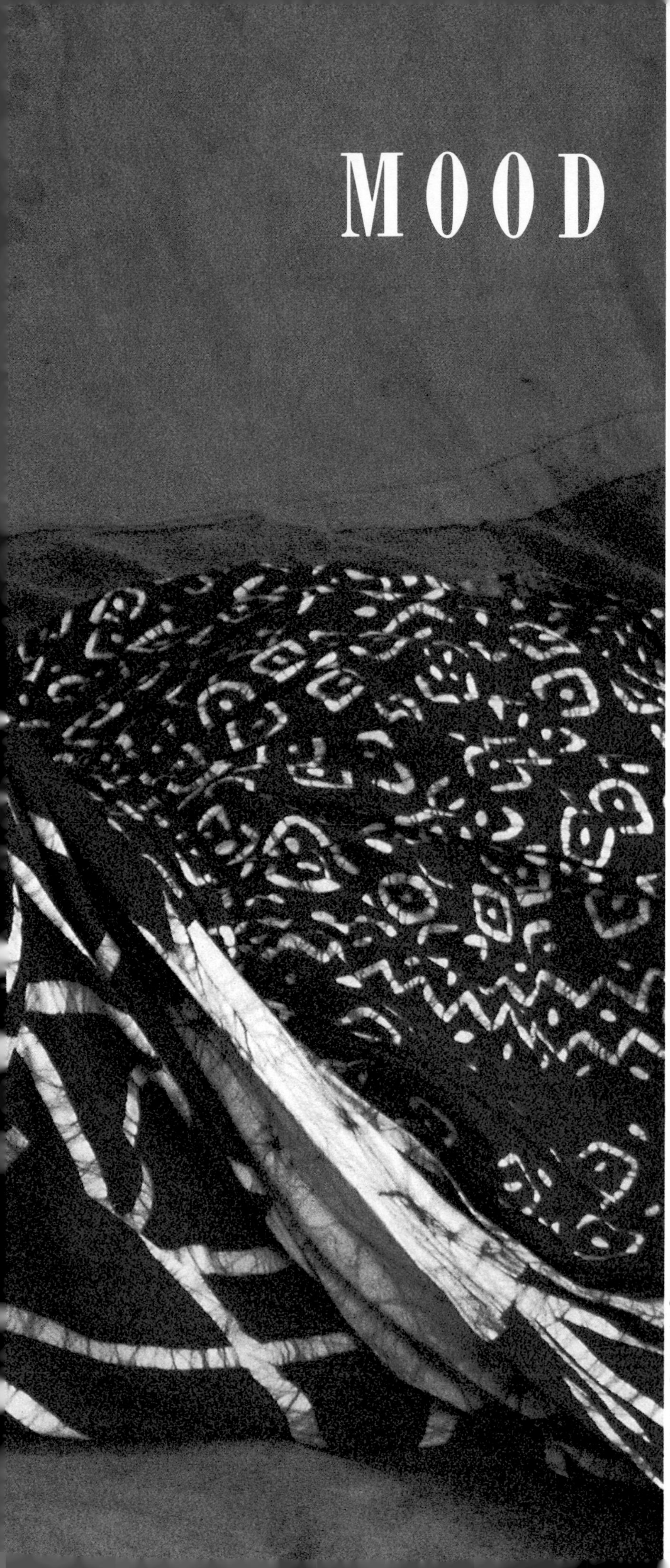

Navy can make a strong statement in summer, with boldly patterned fabric and simple, bold jewellery. With this look you can make the most of your naturally brown limbs, emphatic features, and the healthy gleam of eyes and teeth against your skin. For the best effect the look should be carried right through from head to toe: a coil of turban on the head; plain leather sandals; hoops of silver on the ears; and chunky bands of polished wood on the arms.

It pays to take time to find the right foundation for you or to mix the colours to suit yourself. Make-up created for suntanned skins can work if you are pale brown, and very dark skins may find what they need within theatrical make-up ranges or make-up ranges designed for black skins. For Jane's eye make-up here I used blue, rust and ochre.

'It takes generous amounts of fabric to make a turban that looks impressive and stays in place. This one was shaped from a four-foot length of cloth, wound and twisted round the head and tied in front. See the make-up tips on page 45.' **J F**

Clothes: Comme des Garçons

TECHNICAL TIPS

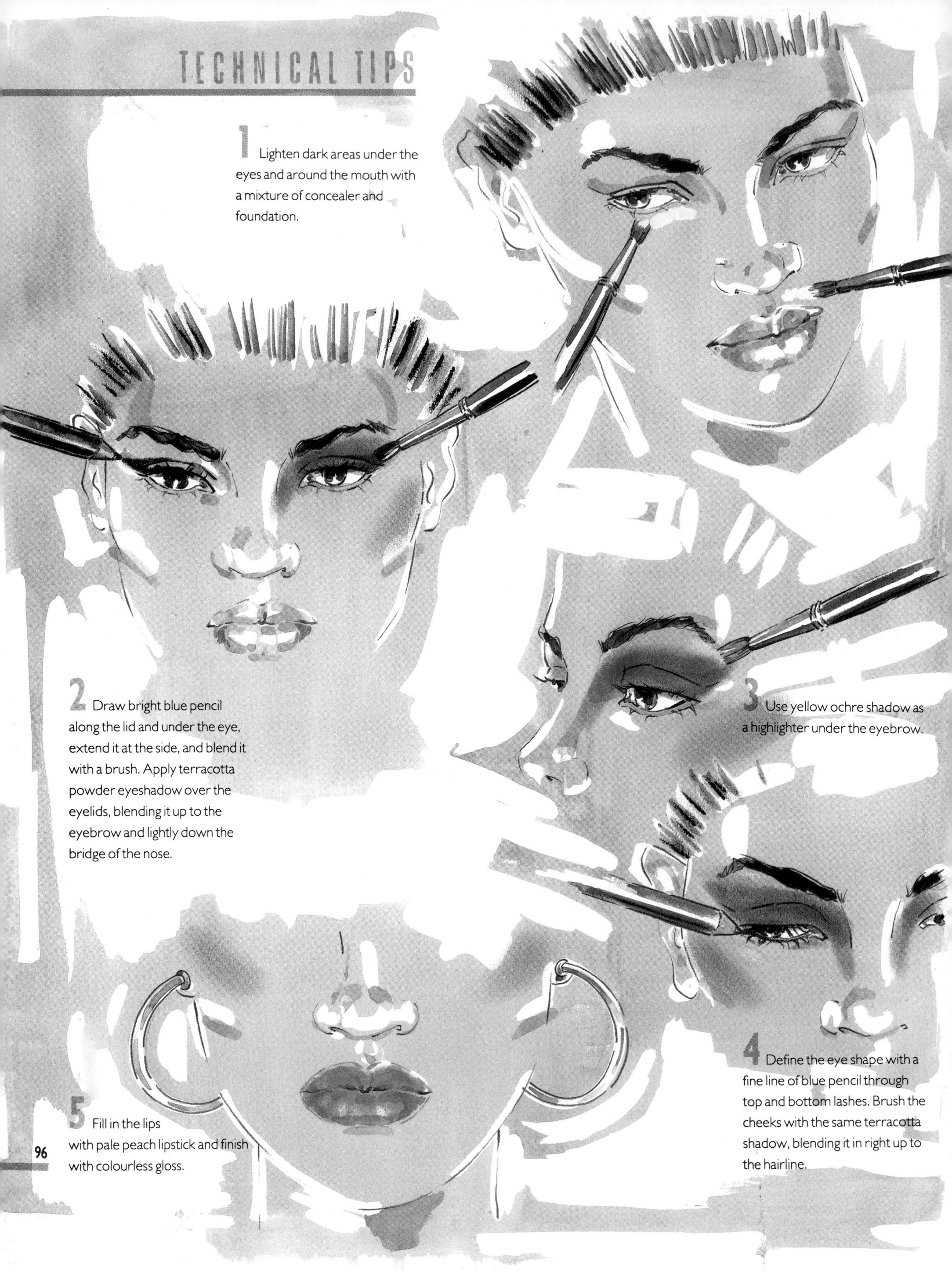

1 Lighten dark areas under the eyes and around the mouth with a mixture of concealer and foundation.

2 Draw bright blue pencil along the lid and under the eye, extend it at the side, and blend it with a brush. Apply terracotta powder eyeshadow over the eyelids, blending it up to the eyebrow and lightly down the bridge of the nose.

3 Use yellow ochre shadow as a highlighter under the eyebrow.

4 Define the eye shape with a fine line of blue pencil through top and bottom lashes. Brush the cheeks with the same terracotta shadow, blending it in right up to the hairline.

5 Fill in the lips with pale peach lipstick and finish with colourless gloss.

A mixture of foundation colours was applied as base. Dark areas around the mouth and under the eyes were lightened with concealer mixed with foundation, then the whole face dusted with transparent powder. Bright blue pencil on the lid and under the eye, extended at the side, was blended with a brush and set with the same face powder. Terracotta powder eyeshadow brushed over the eyelid and into the crease of the eye defines the shape, blended up to the eyebrow and lightly down the bridge of the nose. Yellow ochre shadow was used as a highlighter under the eyebrow. I used black mascara on the lashes and outlined the eye with fine blue pencil through the top and bottom lashes. The same terracotta shadow was brushed on the cheeks as a blusher, and the ochre shadow used to highlight the cheek bones. The lips were filled in with a pale peach lipstick, and finished with colourless gloss.

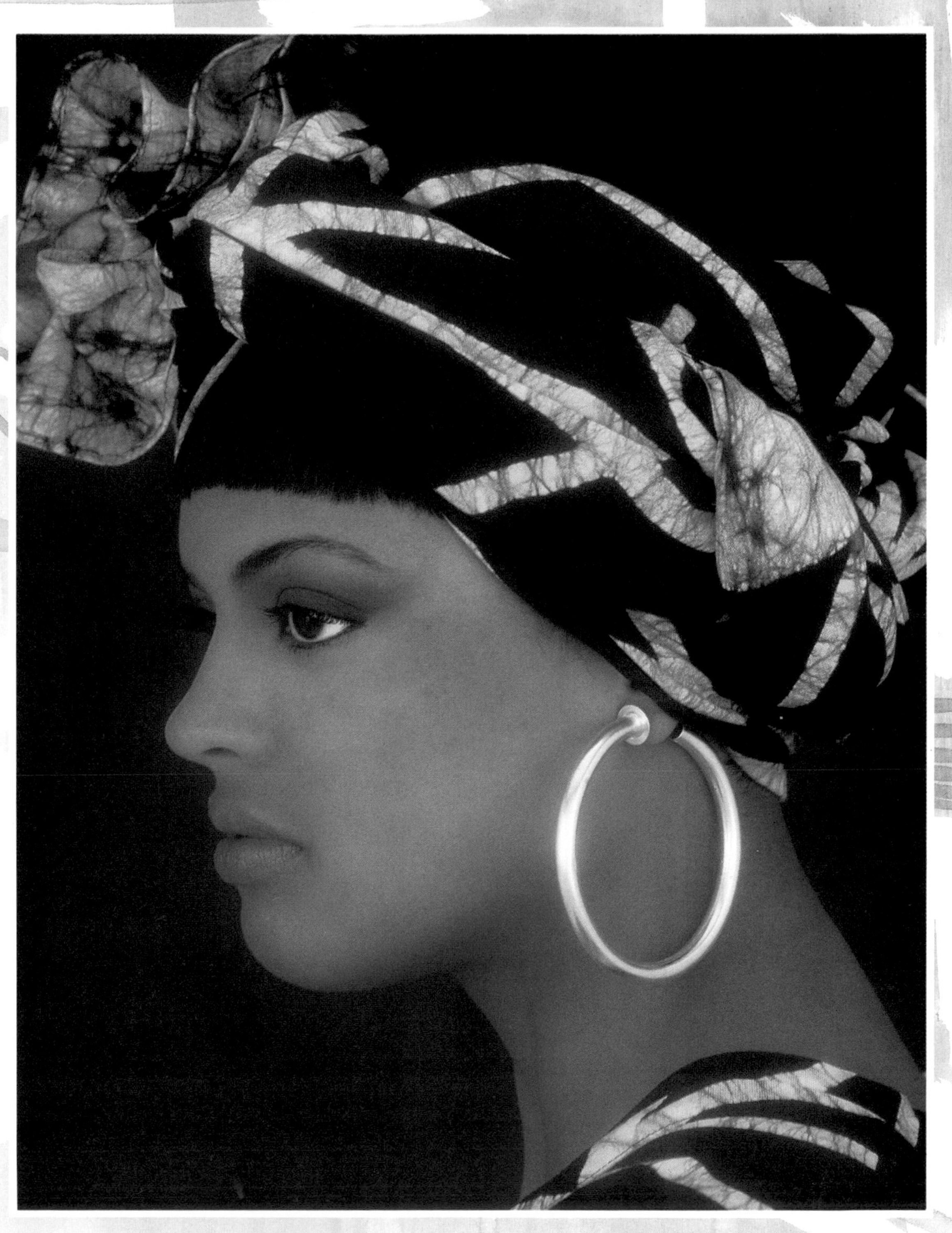

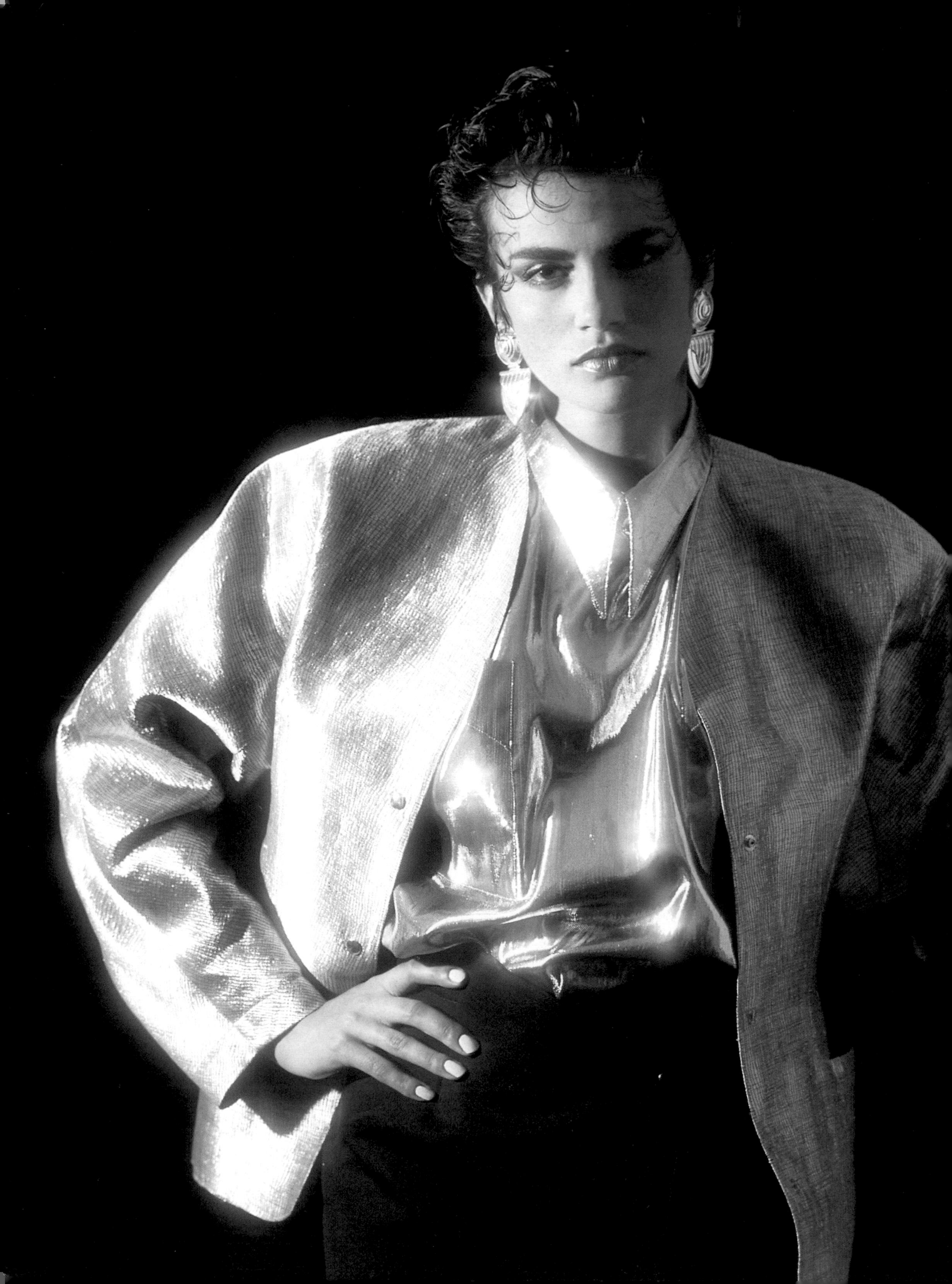

QUICKSILVER

Silver is perfect for evenings when glitter and shine bring the focus of attention your way. But you need to follow through with nails, face and jewellery for maximum impact.

Silver and black is a classic match that can't be bettered. The flamboyant scale of the silvered jacket and shirt is precisely balanced by a narrow black skirt. No other jewellery than the imposing silver earrings is needed.

The metallic theme of the make-up is surprisingly warm. Silver on the eyes gives a seductive glitter, and the full bronze mouth is soft.

'Hair wax was worked through the hair so that it could be slicked back from the face. Then I teased it with a comb into wet-look waves all over the head, pulling out tendrils around the face to add a touch of vulnerability.' **J F**

Suit: Thierry Mugler at Browns · Earrings: Butler & Wilson ·

The base for the silver look is a skin-toned coloured foundation set with a transparent powder. I brushed silver powder eyeshadow all over the upper eyelid and faded it away towards the eyebrow. A line of black cake eyeliner was drawn with a brush along the upper eyelid close to the lashes, and extended slightly beyond the end of the lid. I drew another black line in the eye crease, and smudged it into the sides of the shadow on the upper lid so that the central panel of silver gleams more brightly in contrast. The black is blended away to 'nothing' with a brush towards the eyebrow. A silvery-white powder highlighter was used on the browbone to give extra emphasis. Black mascara completes the eyes. Don't forget to brush out any surplus make-up sticking to your eyebrows and brush them into shape with an old toothbrush or brow-comb. Peach blusher is fluffed on to the cheeks. I chose a metallic bronze lipstick, using a lipbrush to draw a clean outline before filling in.

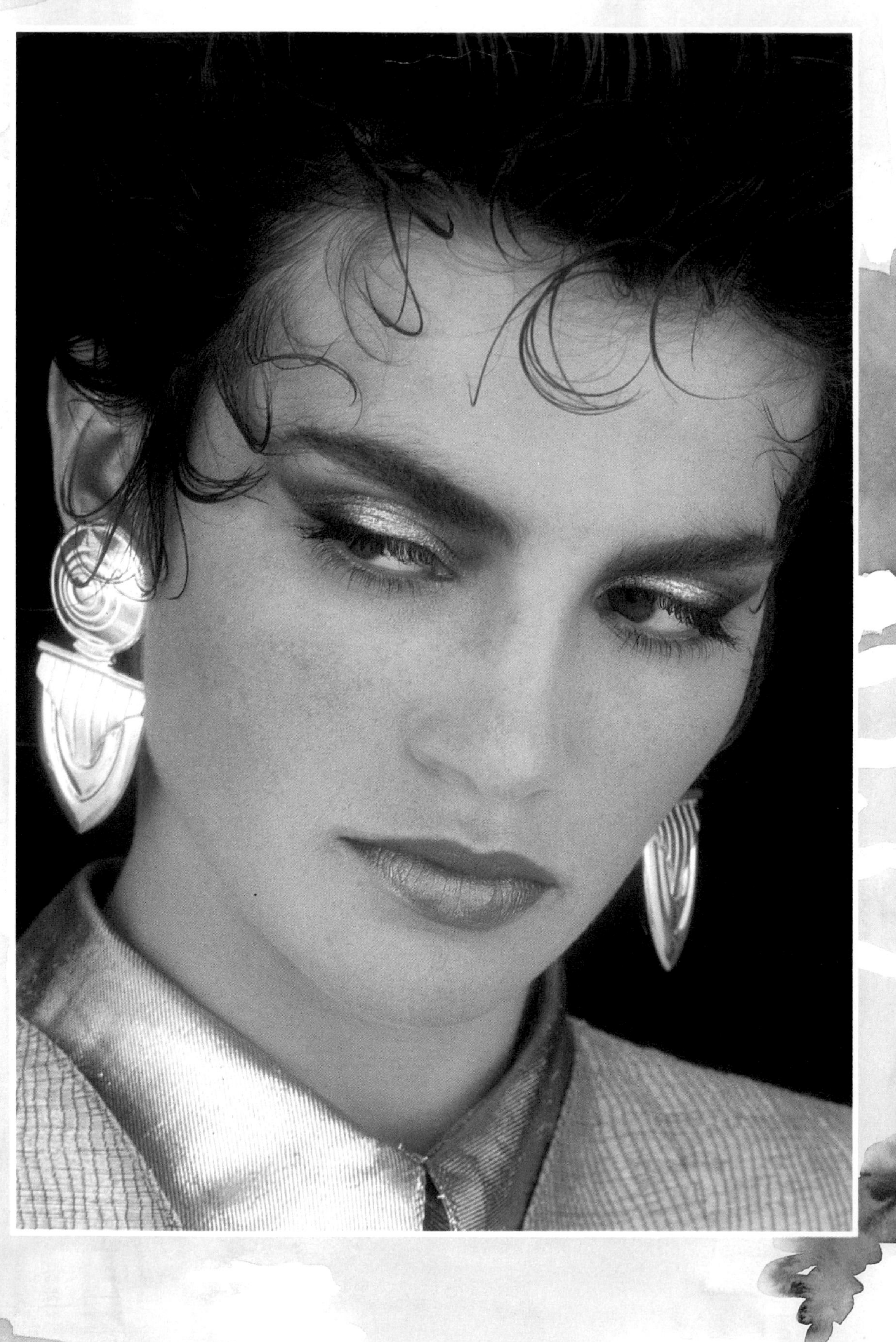

A mixture of foundation colours was applied as base. Dark areas around the mouth and under the eyes were lightened with concealer mixed with foundation, then the whole face dusted with transparent powder. Bright blue pencil on the lid and under the eye, extended at the side, was blended with a brush and set with the same face powder. Terracotta powder eyeshadow brushed over the eyelid and into the crease of the eye defines the shape, blended up to the eyebrow and lightly down the bridge of the nose. Yellow ochre shadow was used as a highlighter under the eyebrow. I used black mascara on the lashes and outlined the eye with fine blue pencil through the top and bottom lashes. The same terracotta shadow was brushed on the cheeks as a blusher, and the ochre shadow used to highlight the cheek bones. The lips were filled in with a pale peach lipstick, and finished with colourless gloss.

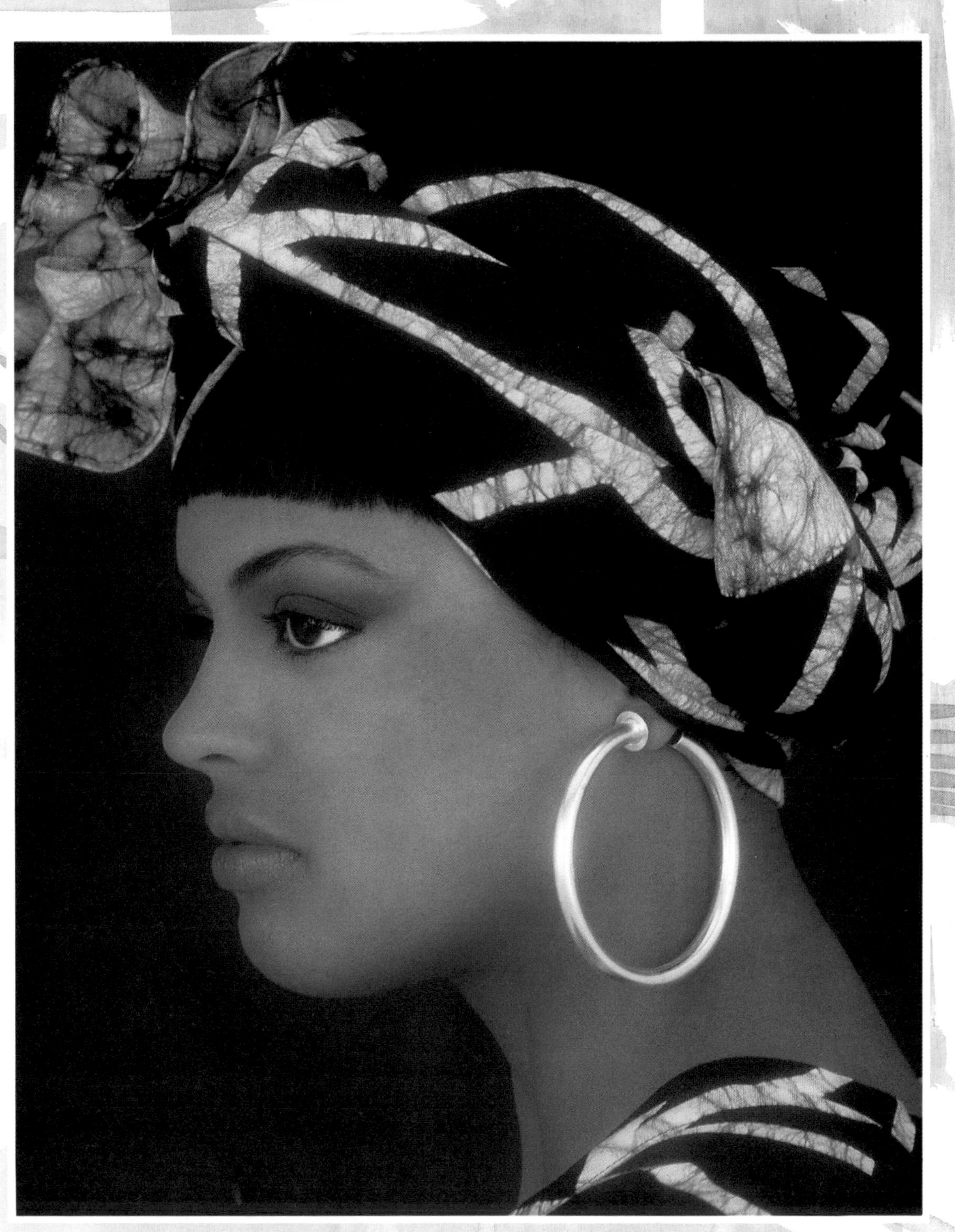

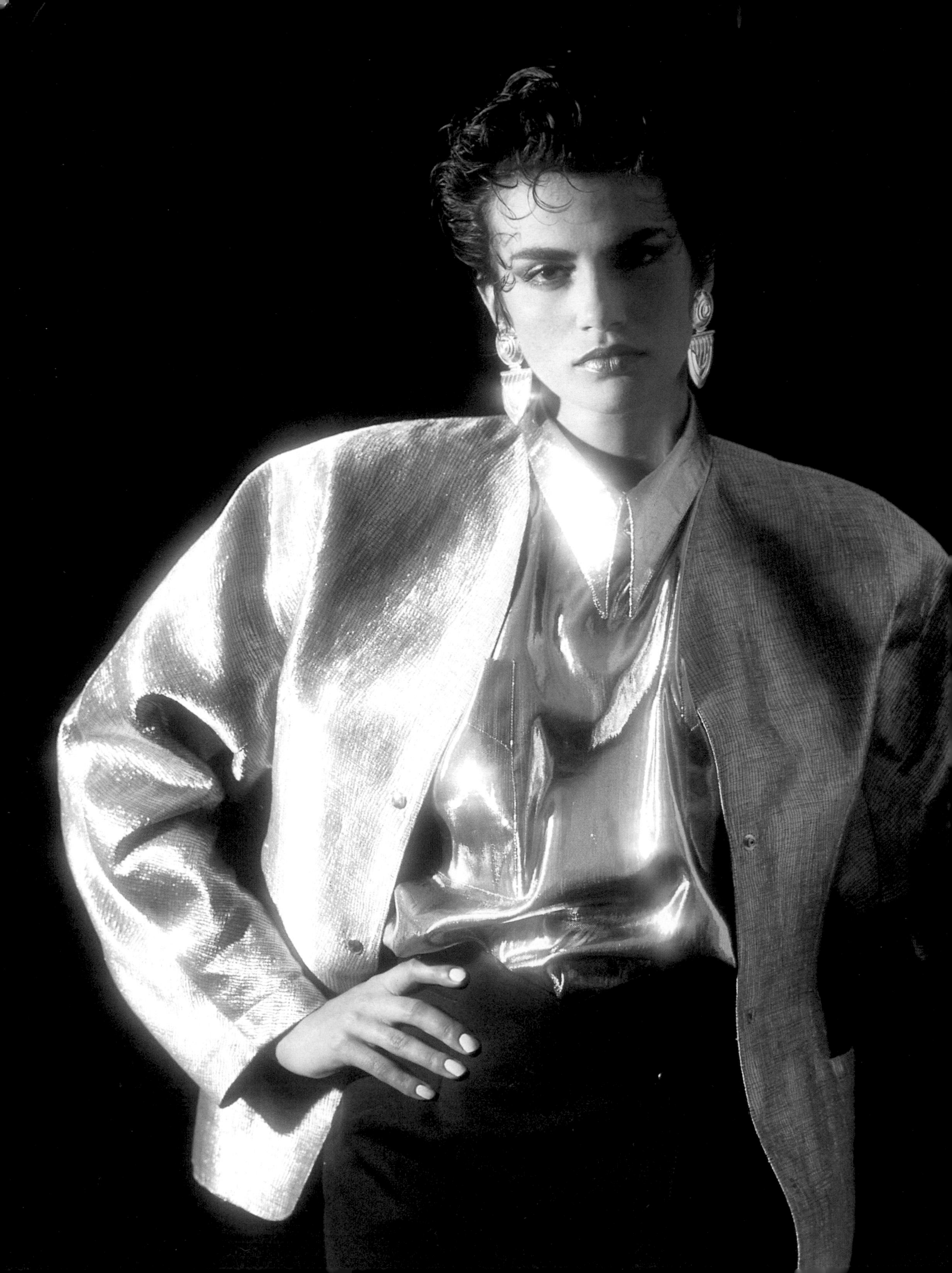

TECHNICAL TIPS

1 After applying silver powder eyeshadow, draw a black cake eyeliner along the upper lid and also into the socket line.

2 Use a silvery-white highlighter on the browbone for extra emphasis.

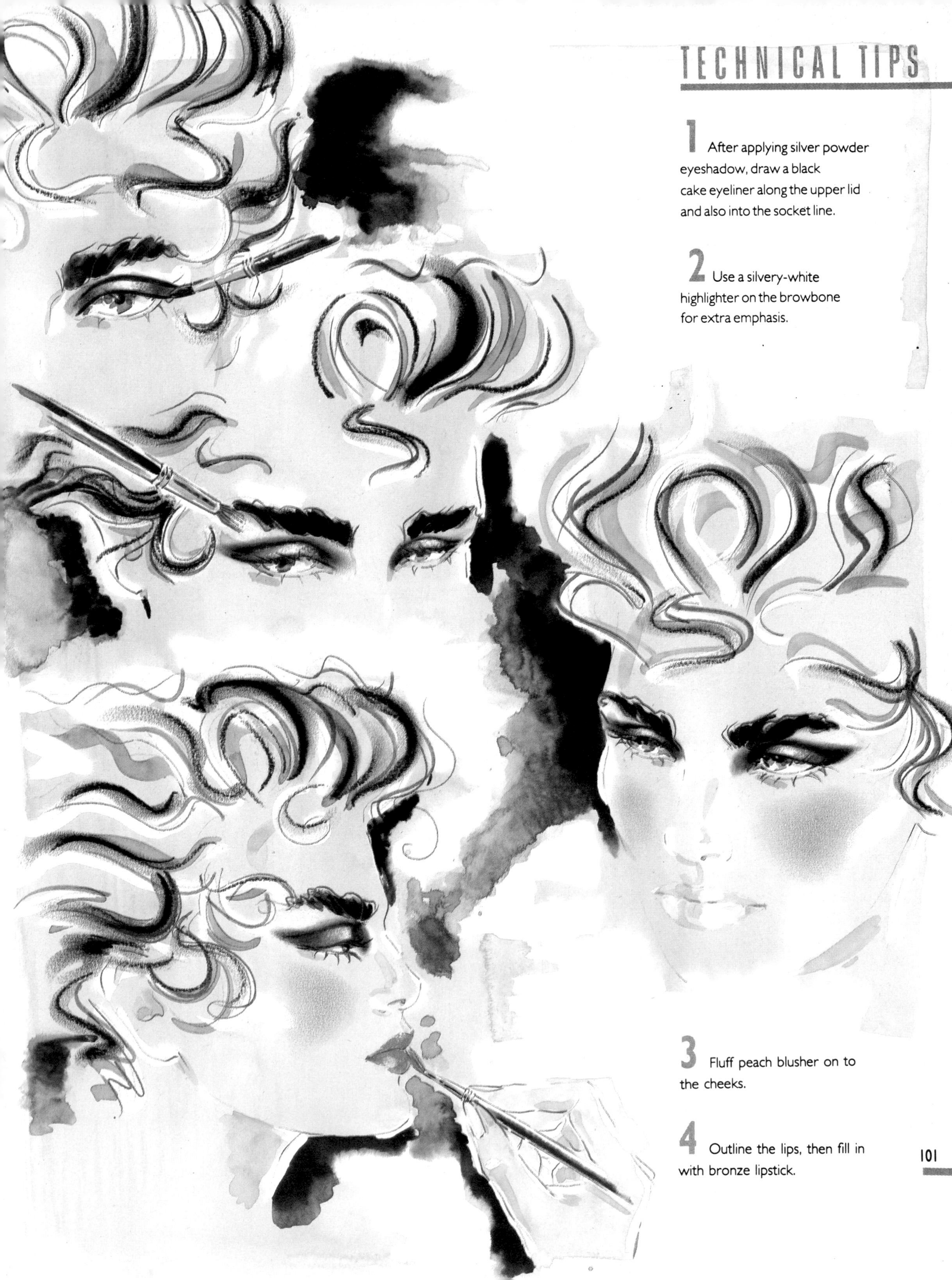

3 Fluff peach blusher on to the cheeks.

4 Outline the lips, then fill in with bronze lipstick.

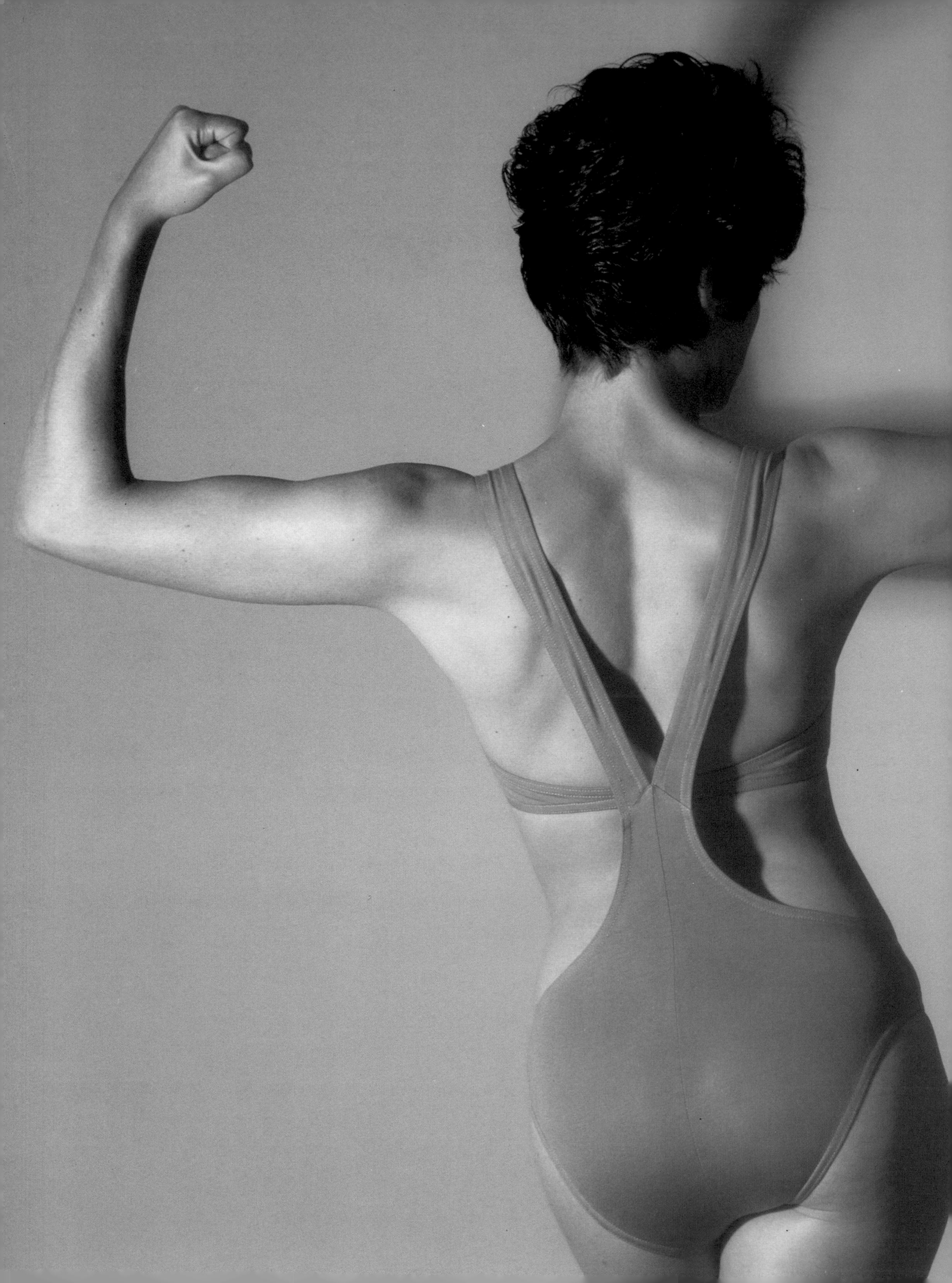

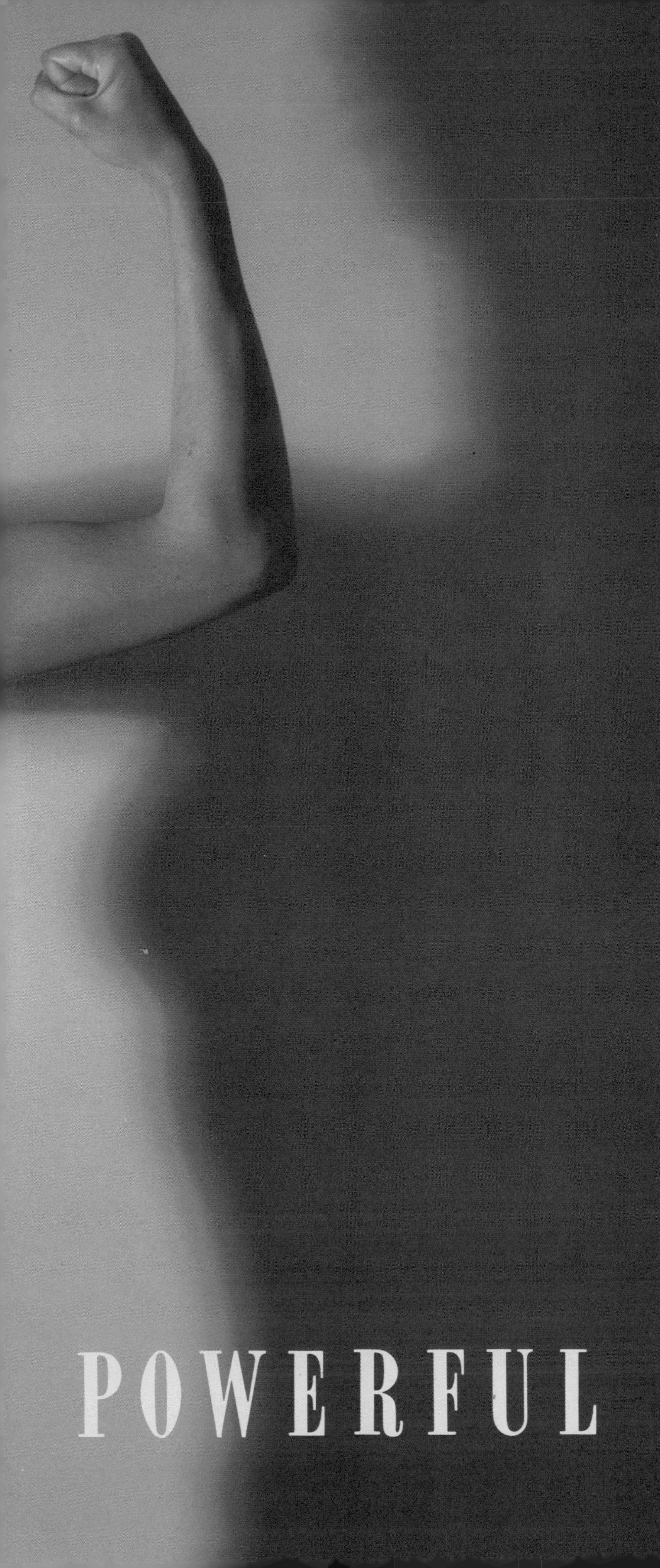

BRUNETTE

Costume: Azzedine Alaïa at Joseph Tricot · Sunglasses: Issey Miyake · Towel: Descamps ·

Peach is a skin-toned colour and can therefore look very natural. Against the olive skin of a dark-haired girl it creates the healthy glow that goes with feeling fit, working out, and being in tip-top condition. A sun-lover goes for the minimal look, a one-piece swimming costume, cut to flatter every sleek curve of a well-exercised body. The only accessories you need are a towel, sunglasses and, of course, your sun tan preparations.

Sun and make-up don't mix. If you want to look your best for cocktail-sipping in the shade you can add the bare essentials of colour – something that you can whisk off quickly before diving in the water or stretching out in the sun.

'To give the hair a natural-looking bounce it was blowdried, lifting it at the roots with a brush to give fullness. A little sun cream was stroked through with the hands so that it could be pulled into spiky fronds, and also to protect the hair from the sun. 'Draw lines' were made at the back with a wide-toothed comb.' **J F**

POWERFUL PEACH

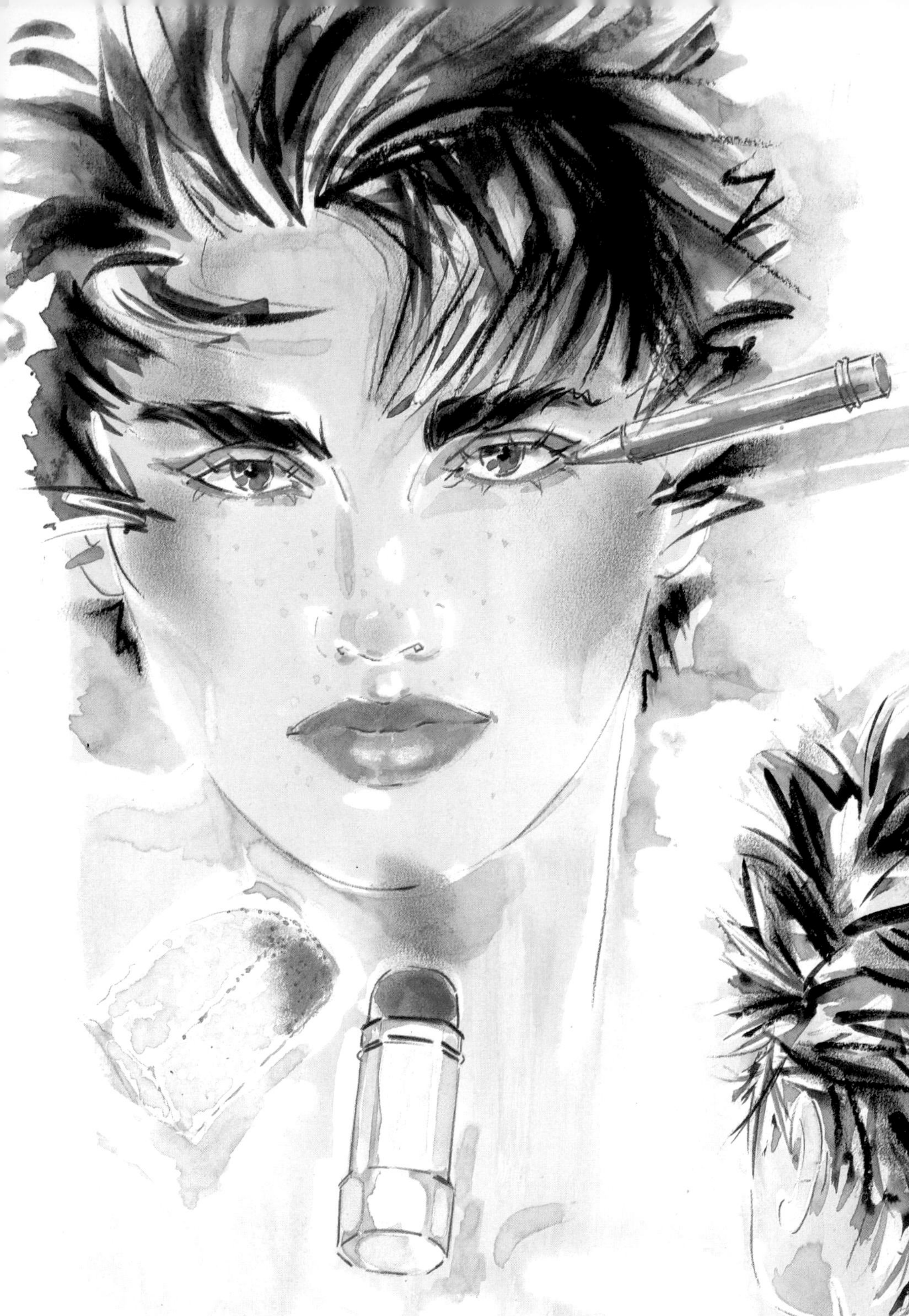

1 Apply cream blusher in a deep peach with a sponge on cheeks, temples and very lightly on nose and chin.

2 Draw sea-green kohl pencil on the inner rim of your lower lid.

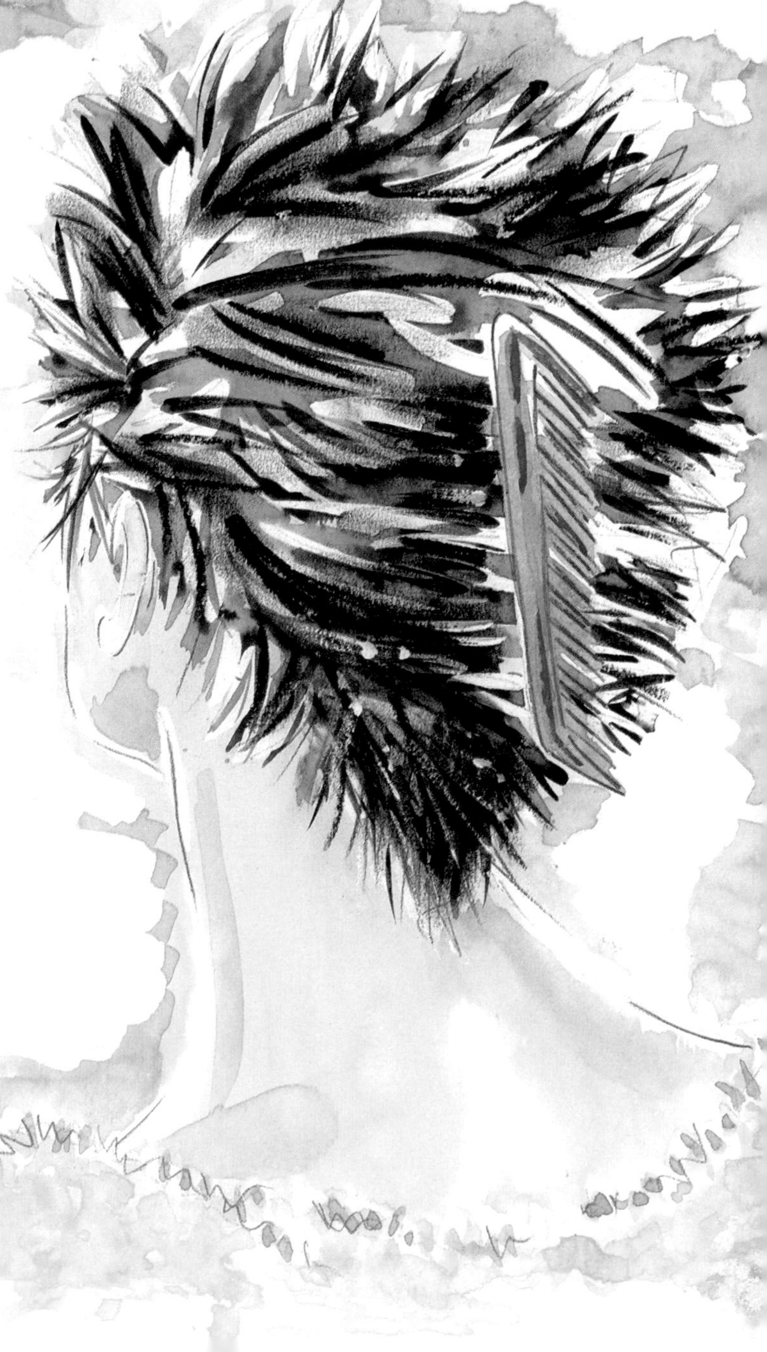

3 Draw lines through your hair with a wide-toothed comb after stroking a little sun cream through it.

If you are going to spend time out in the sun, dispense with foundation, and invest in a good sun cream instead. A high-factor sun block will allow you to tan, but will filter out the burning rays. Cream blusher in a deep peach colour applied with a sponge on cheeks, temples and very lightly on your nose and chin, makes you look as if you've had a touch of the sun already, and is easily wiped off when the sunbathing starts. Not much eye make-up here, except for sea-green pencil kohl on the inner rim of your lower lid. Lipstick can be as bright and strong as you wish — unlike a lot of eye make-up it looks good in the sun. I chose a colour which exactly matches the bathing costume.

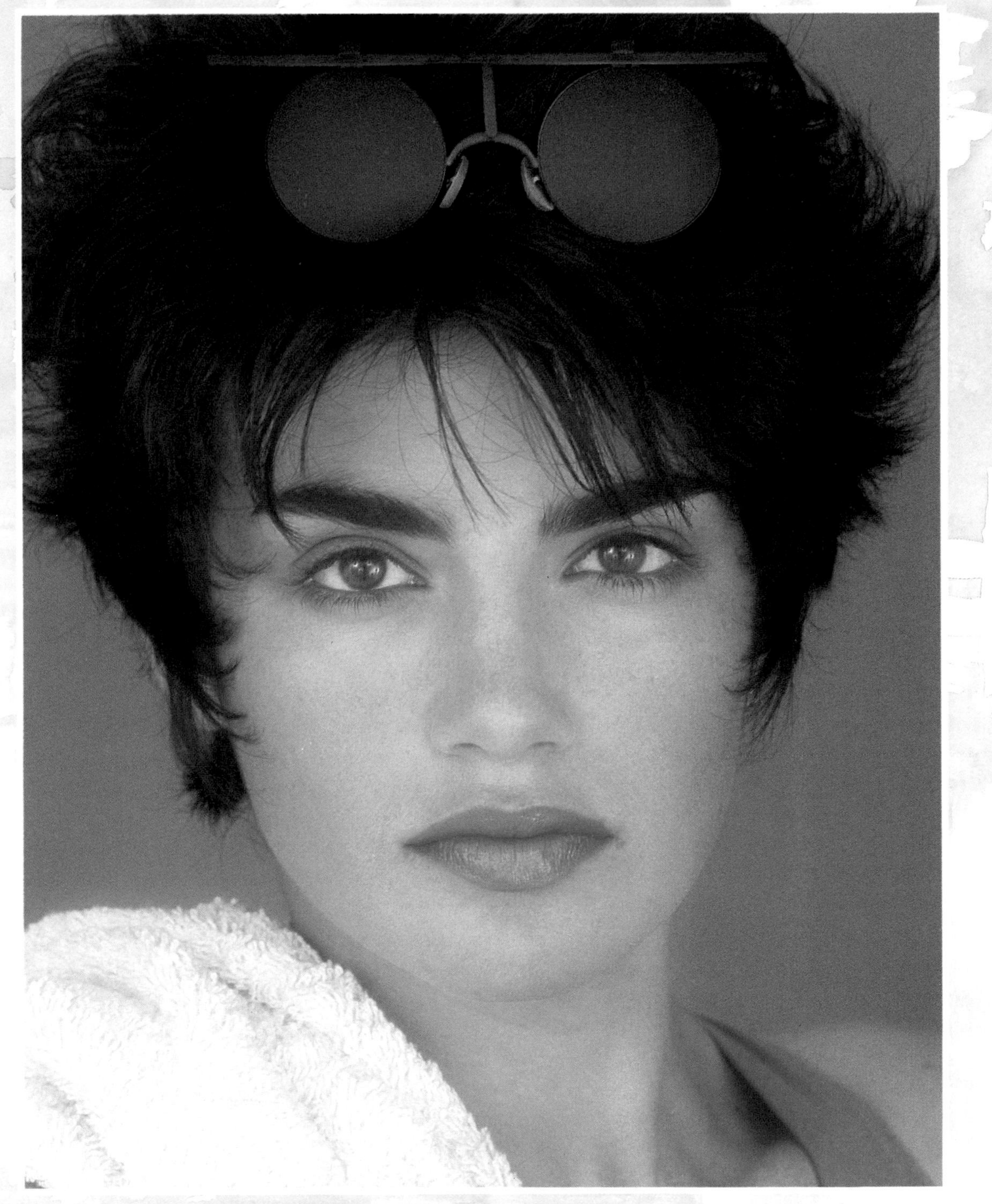

VIOLETTA

Purple is traditionally regarded as a royal colour. Set against pale skin and black hair the effect is undeniably compelling. The gorgeous richness of the fabric of this simple dress needs nothing to break the long inky fall. All detail is concentrated round the head: an imaginative hat of gold-swirled pink, and the delicately worked gold and purple earring. This is a look that is aristocratic and impressive.

The make-up I designed to complement the clothes is a flow of lilacs and purples on eyes and lips, melting into the paleness of the face.

'I styled the hair with gel, so that when the hat was placed at the correct angle, waves could be flicked up around the brim, and soft curls combed out round the cheeks and ears.' **J F**

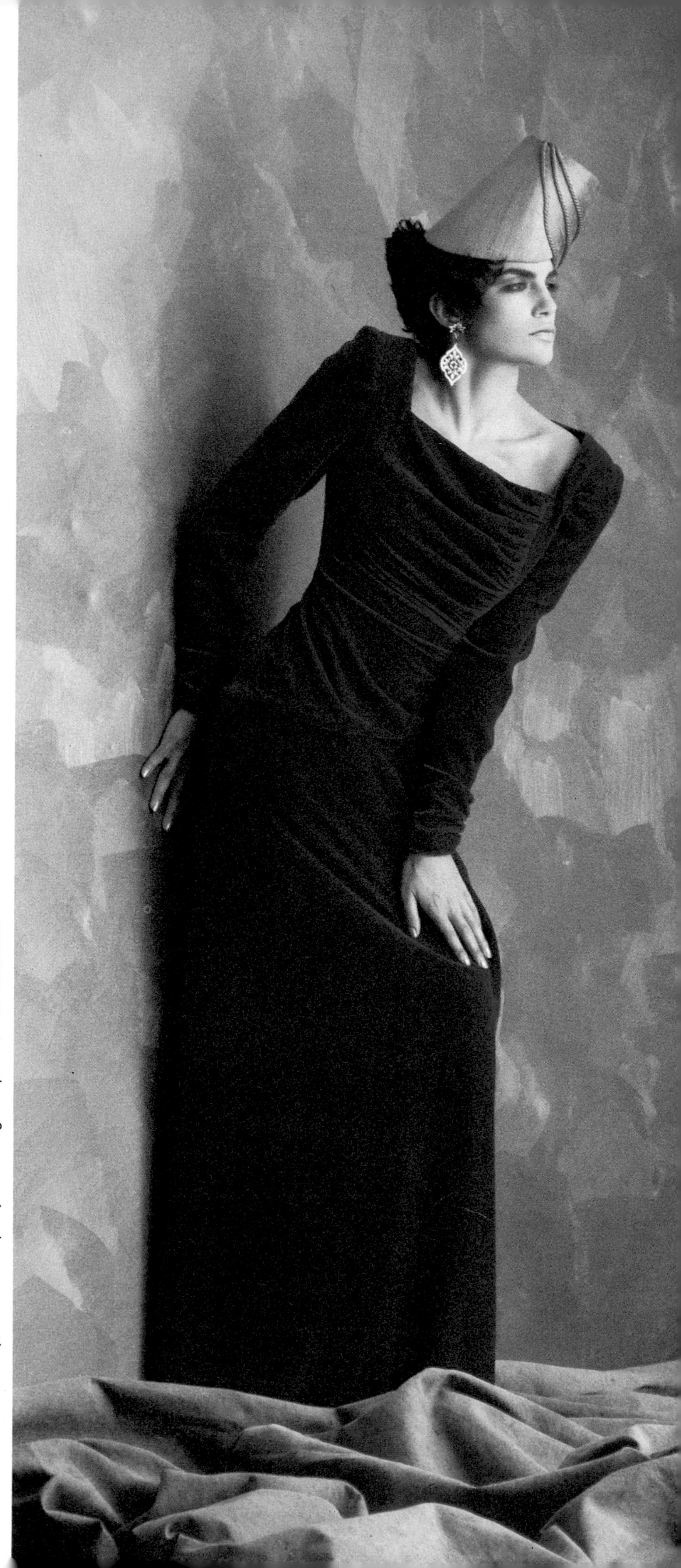

Dress: Murray Arbeid · Hat: Stephen Jones · Earrings: Dinny Hall · Shoes: Maud Frizon ·

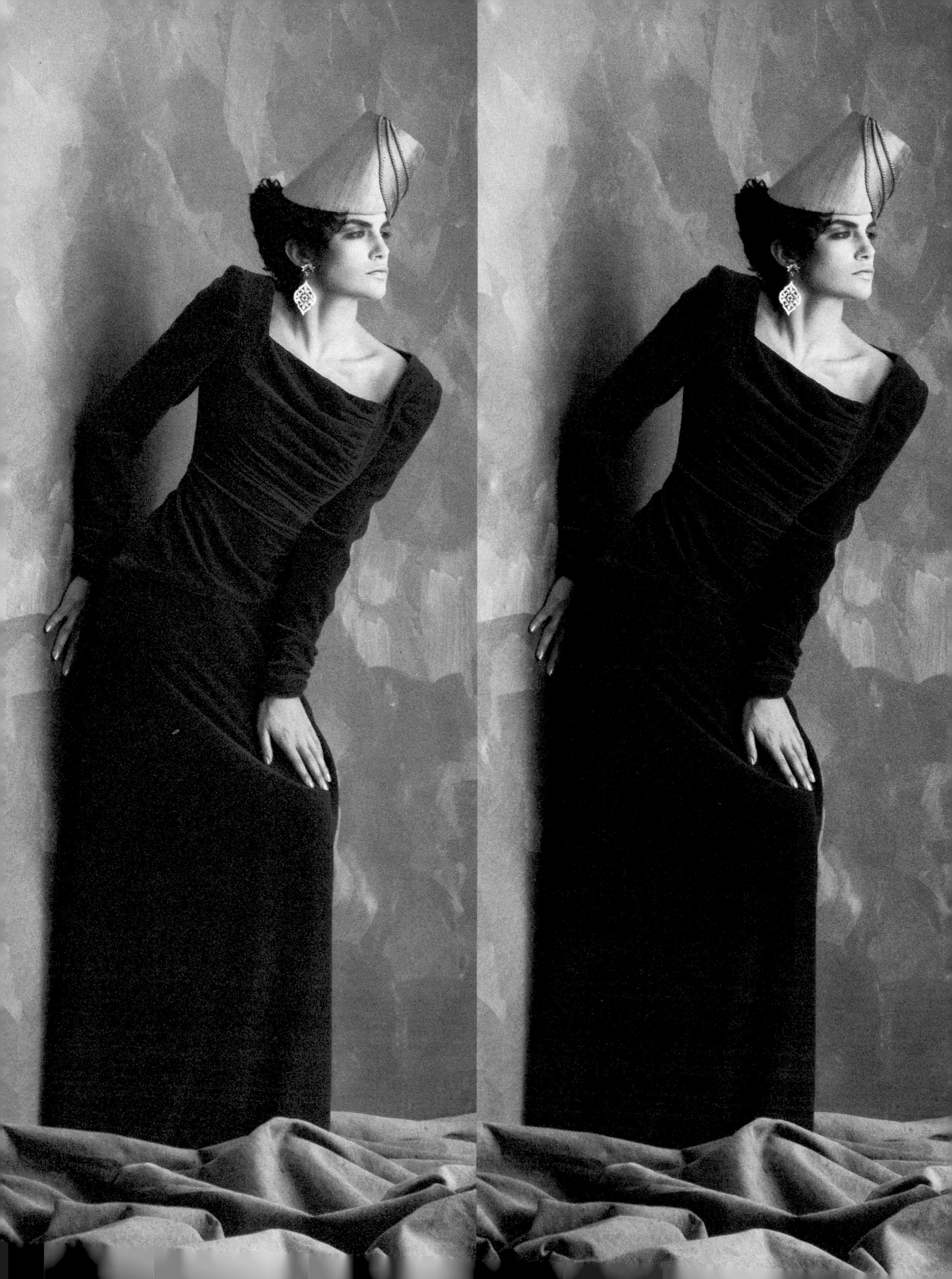

Pale foundation was applied with a sponge and well blended so that Debbie's own warmer skin tone did not show through, then I set the base with face powder. Dark purple eyeshadow was stroked into the crease of the eye. I drew a line of violet eye pencil along the upper lid close to the lashes, then another along the lower lid so that the two lines met to form a 'V' at the outer corner of the eye. Pale lavender shadow was brushed on to the upper eyelid and browbone as a highlighter. I mixed lavender shadow with pink blusher and used them as a blusher, brushed on temple and cheek. Purple mascara for the lashes and violet kohl pencil on the inner rim of the lower lid finished the eyes. The mouth was outlined very lightly with a pink pencil and filled in with lavender lipstick.

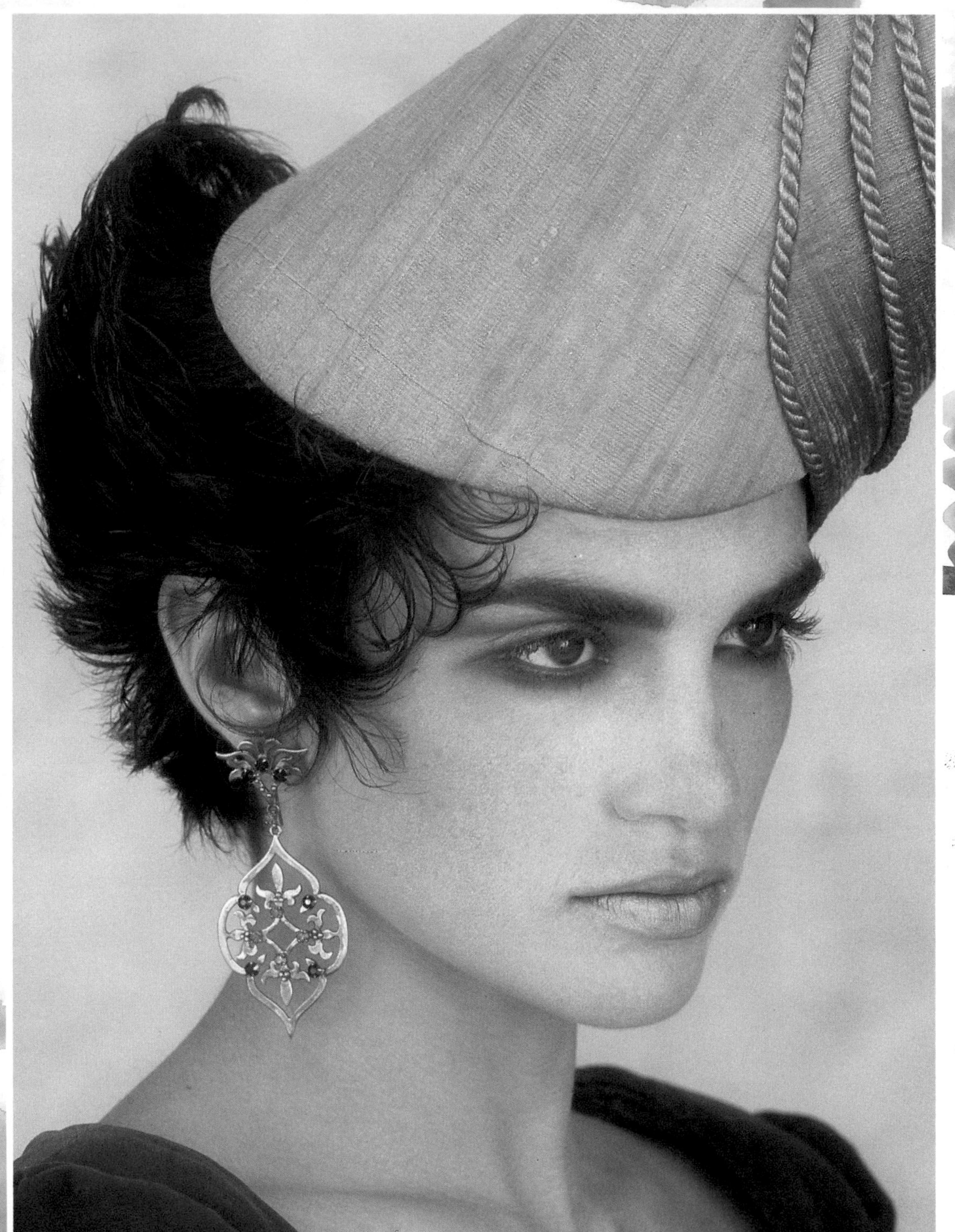

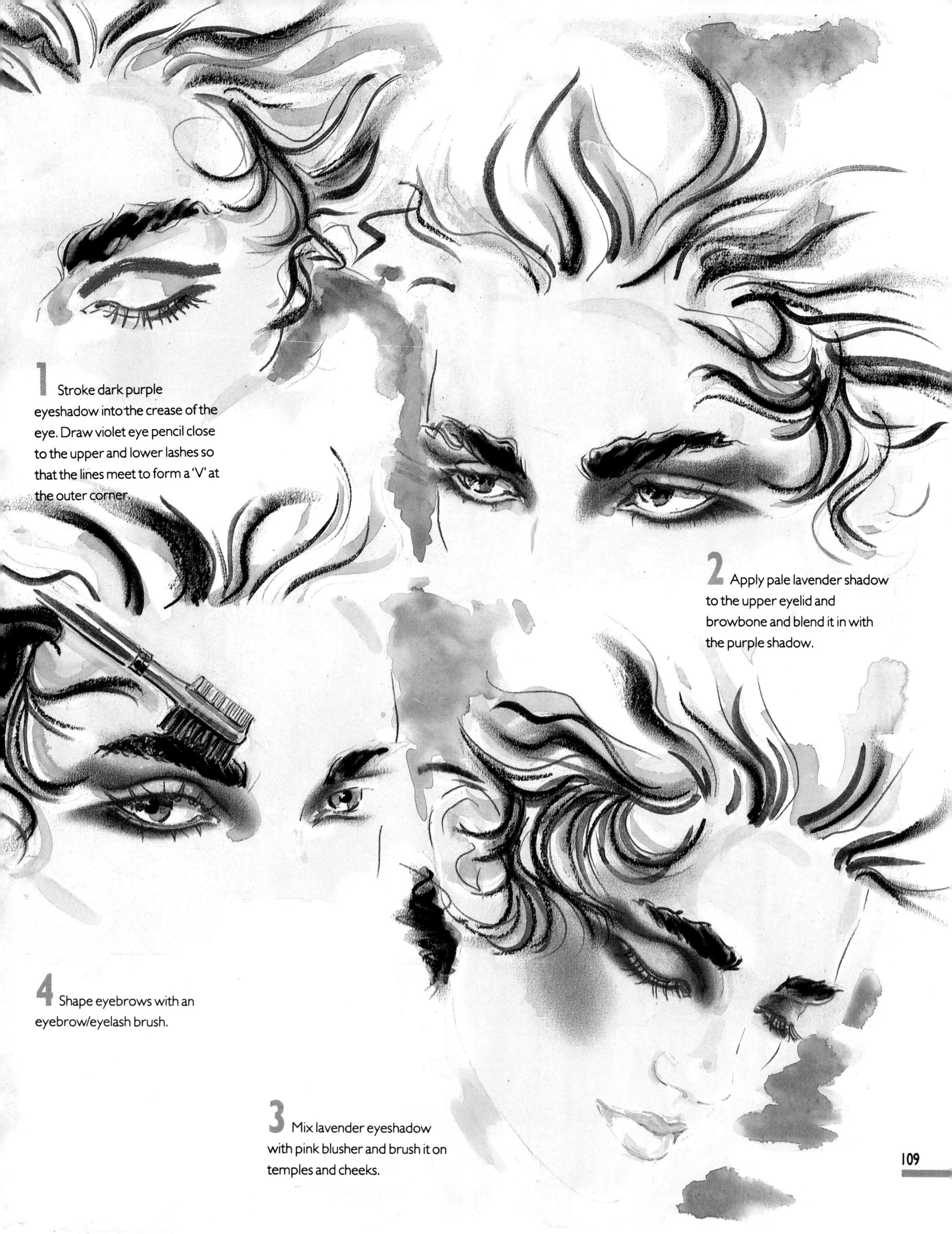

1 Stroke dark purple eyeshadow into the crease of the eye. Draw violet eye pencil close to the upper and lower lashes so that the lines meet to form a 'V' at the outer corner.

2 Apply pale lavender shadow to the upper eyelid and browbone and blend it in with the purple shadow.

4 Shape eyebrows with an eyebrow/eyelash brush.

3 Mix lavender eyeshadow with pink blusher and brush it on temples and cheeks.

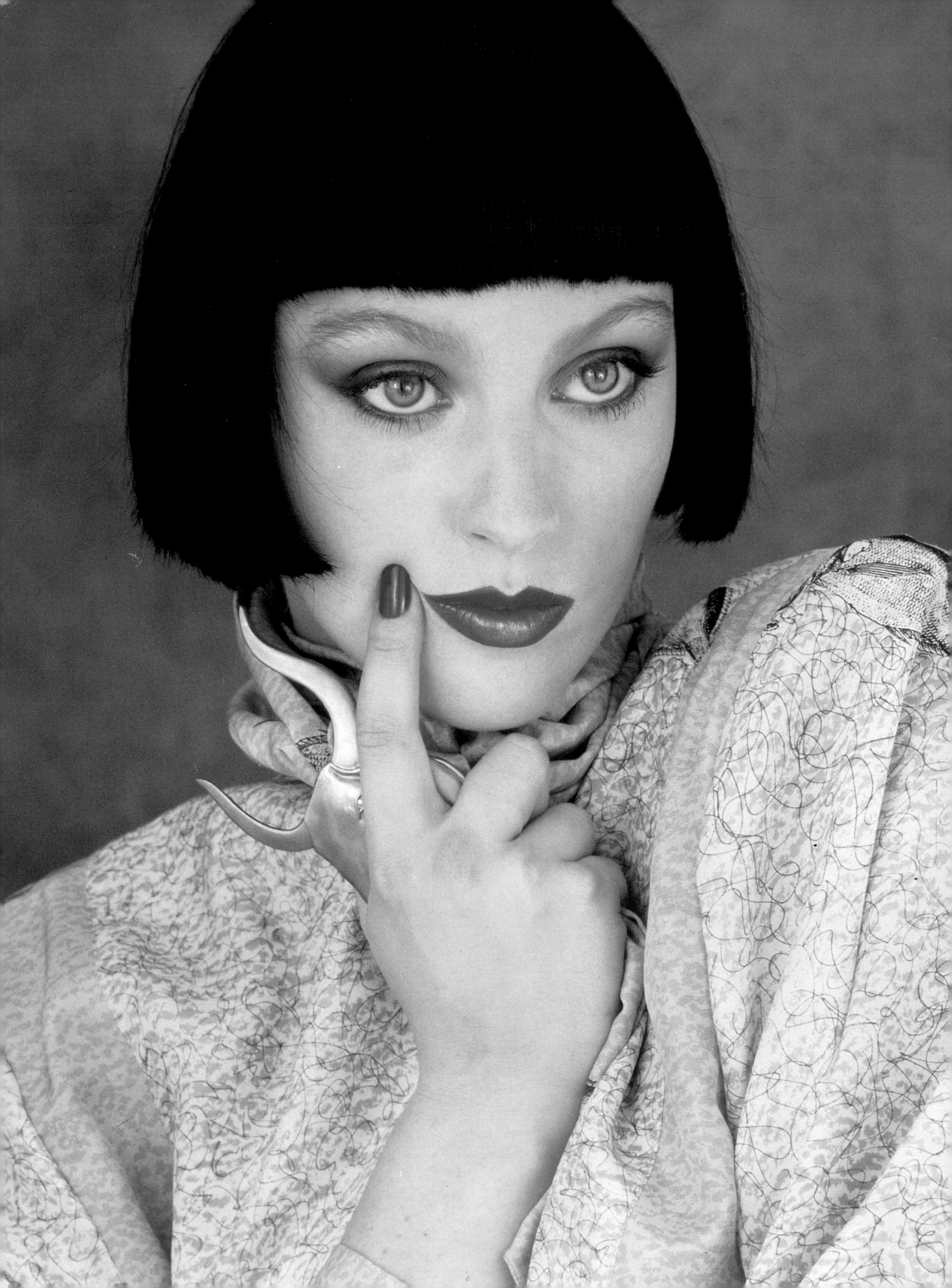

INDEX

ACKNOWLEDGMENTS

The author and publishers would like to thank the following companies for their assistance in lending clothes and accessories for photography:

JACKET PHOTOGRAPH
Dress and hat, Wendy Dagworthy

PAGE 11
Towel, Descamps

PAGES 22-3
Clothes, Crolla; shoes, Manolo Blahnik

PAGES 26-7
Shirt specially coloured by Swanky Modes; jewellery, Gary Wright & Sheila Teague

PAGES 28-9
T-shirt dress, Comme des Garçons

PAGES 35-40
Rings, Monty Don; mirror, Conran

PAGE 41
Dress, Betty Jackson; jewellery, Gary Wright & Sheila Teague

PAGES 50-3
Clothes, Joseph Tricot

PAGES 54-7
Clothes, Joseph pour la maison; earrings, Butler & Wilson; brooch, Monty Don; bangles, Gary Wright & Sheila Teague

PAGES 58-61
Suede dress, Maxfield Parrish; jacket, John McIntyre; brooch, Monty Don; earrings, Gary Wright & Sheila Teague

PAGES 62-5
Wedding dress and veil, Tatters

PAGES 66-9
Clothes, Sonia Rykiel at Browns; shoes, Maud Frizon; earrings, Butler & Wilson

PAGES 70-3
Suit, Sonia Rykiel at Browns; scarf, Whistles; shoes, Maud Frizon; jewellery, Monty Don

PAGES 74-7
Camisole top, skirt and hat, Ralph Lauren; coat-dress, Margaret Howell

PAGES 78-81
Pink suit, Gaultier at Browns; orange shirt and bra top, Whistles; earrings, Detail

PAGES 82-5
Clothes, Betty Jackson: hat, Viv Knowland; brooch, Monty Don

PAGES 86-9
Clothes, Ralph Lauren; plimsolls, Whistles

PAGES 90-3 (AND PAGE 6)
Dress, Whistles; coat, Gaultier at Browns; earrings, Monty Don

PAGES 94-7
Clothes, Comme des Garçons; jewellery, Gary Wright & Sheila Teague

PAGES 98-101
Suit, Thierry Mugler at Browns; earrings, Butler & Wilson

PAGES 102-5
Costume, Azzedine Alaïa at Joseph Tricot; sunglasses, Issey Miyake; towel, Descamps

PAGES 106-9
Dress, Murray Arbeid; hat, Stephen Jones; shoes, Maud Frizon; earrings, Dinny Hall